More comments from the industry about Marijuana, Gateway To Health:

"Billions of dollars' worth of pharmaceuticals are based on opium and cocaine, yet the active ingredients of marijuana are shunned. If just 5% of Werner's claims regarding the clinical benefits of cannabinoids are true, why are governments and drug manufacturers so intransigent about marijuana? Can 'pot' be more dangerous—and less beneficial—than legally distributed Oxycontin, ephedrine, Percocet or Valium?"
—Laurie Garrett, author of *I Heard The Sirens Scream: How Americans Responded to the 9/11 and Anthrax Attacks*

"Clint Werner argues forcefully that the health benefits of marijuana far exceed its dangers. Much of the evidence is preliminary, but it adds up to a call for professional, large-scale scientific research to access this ancient and ever more popular herb."
—Robert Bazell, author *Her-2: The Making of Herceptin, a Revolutionary Treatment for Breast Cancer*

"Loaded with footnotes and packed with information, *Marijuana Gateway to Health* will teach any skeptic how medical marijuana heals people."
—High Times Magazine

"If government policy is ever based on science instead of Big Lies, this book contains the science it will be based upon. Buy a copy before you get old. Buy a copy for your doctor!"
—Michale and Michelle Aldrich, The Aldrich Archives, San Francisco

"Clint Werner's book, *Marijuana Gateway To Health* is packed with scientific revelations about cannabis—a real eye opener and a must read. It is refreshing to see the truth!"
—Brad Lane, Executive Producer, Cannabis Planet TV

"The compilation of scientific studies in this book is just superb. I can't wait to see how *Marijuana Gateway To Health* changes the world as we know it"
—Angela Fairless, LaRoach.com

D0816985

"Clint Werner's *Marijuana: Gateway to Health* sets a new milestone in the understanding of marijuana as medicine. This book is a masterpiece—clearly written, well documented, and it pushes back against the ill-conceived propaganda against these useful plants. Any skeptic is well advised to read this book before voicing an opinion. I highly recommend this book !"
—Paul Stamets, author *Growing Gourmet and Medicinal Mushrooms* and *Mycellium Running*

"*Marijuana: Gateway to Health* is a refreshingly readable book that engages the reader from page one. Werner brings to life the story of how marijuana's medical benefits have been discovered, covering all the bases and putting clinical studies into their proper, broader perspective. A terrific book with heart and soul."
—Ellen Komp, editor *The Emperor Wears No Clothes*

"Clint Werner demonstrates numerous qualities of medicinal cannabis with well-documented research and dispels myth after myth. *Marijuana Gateway to Health* delves into everything from Alzheimer's to the War on Drugs with important details on monumental discoveries about the endocannabinoid system and how it can prevent disease and pain. If you want to know about medical marijuana today, this is the best source of information. I keep my copy on my desk!"
—Jorge Cervantes, author *Marijuana Horticulture*, photographer

"*Marijuana Gateway to Health* blends a clear and concise overview of the science supporting cannabis as medicine with an engaging account of the politics of prohibition that still keeps it from patients. Werner shows just how cruel and counterproductive federal marijuana policy is. This book should be required reading for all medical professionals, elected officials, and everyone interested in health and wellness."
—Andrew Weil, M.D. author *Spontaneous Healing and Spontaneous Laughter*

"*Marijuana Gateway to Health* documents important and hitherto under-reported scientific discoveries and developments concerning the endocannabinoid system and how it influences health and wellness."
—Morris Schambelan, MD, Professor Emeritus of Medicine University of California San Francisco

MARIJUANA
GATEWAY
TO
HEALTH

MARIJUANA
GATEWAY
TO
HEALTH

HOW CANNABIS PROTECTS US FROM
CANNER AND ALZHEIMER'S DISEASE

CLINT WERNER

DACHSTAR PRESS
SAN FRANCISCO

Disclaimer

The contents of this book, all text, graphics, images, studies and information are for informational purposes only. The content is not meant to be a substitute for professional medical advice, diagnosis, or treatment. Please do not disregard professional medical advice or delay seeking it because of something you have read in this book.

This information is not meant to prevent, alleviate, or cure any disease or disorder. Always seek the advice of a physician, doctor of chiropractic, or other qualified health provider with any questions you may have regarding a medical condition.

The purpose of this book is to complement, amplify, and supplement other text. You are urged to read all the available material, learn as much as possible, and tailor the information to your individual needs.

Neither the publisher nor the author shall be liable or responsible for any loss or damage allegedly arising from any information or suggestion within these pages or on our websites. Further, if you suspect that you have a medical problem, we urge you to seek professional medical help.

ISBN: 978-0-9834261-8-9
LCCN: 2011931944

Published by
Dachstar Press
P.O. Box 460681
San Francisco, California 94146-0681

URL: www.marijuanagatewaytohealth.com

Printed in the United States of America

THIS BOOK IS DEDICATED TO my parents, Lee and Mary Werner, for making my education their top priority; and to all those unjustly imprisoned for using, growing or selling marijuana, represented by: Mollie Fry, Dale Schafer, Marc Emery and Eddy Lepp.

Contents

Contents

INTRODUCTION

I WROTE THIS BOOK AFTER learning of the growing number of scientific studies which reveal that cannabinoids, the unique compounds found in marijuana, have powerful anti-tumor activity and that they guard the brain from the type of damage that results from toxicity, injury and aging. As more and more of these research reports were published in peer-reviewed journals, they were ignored by the mainstream media, treated as an amusing joke, or reported on sporadically without this important data being pulled together to make the logical assertion that using marijuana is good for human health. Science is a tool we use to understand the world around us. It is the most efficient way we have to separate belief from reality and what the science says about marijuana is that using it regularly will reduce your chances of developing an impressive number of serious illnesses.

The "Eureka!" moment for me, the point at which I knew I had to write *this* book, came after hearing a radio report of a study which found that smoking marijuana significantly reduced the brain damage caused by binge drinking alcohol. As I gathered together research reports I turned to the Pubmed website, which was like hitting a jack pot. I found study after study—amazing research—which few in the general public, or the medical field were aware of. The conclusions were nothing short of mind blowing—cannabinoids inhibit tumor growth, THC kills tumors, THC triggers healthy brain cell production, CBD could delay the onset of diabetes. I would research and write and then walk around the house with my head in my hands, hoping it would not explode in amazement. It was hard to keep up with this body of evidence that was expanding faster than I could document it. After completing the manuscript, there was the frustration of new research being published that showed children with residual brain tumors saw no progression of growth in the cancer while they were inhaling marijuana or that cannabinoids might delay the onset of Huntington's disease better than any known treatment.

I've written this book to serve as an accessible and comprehensive guide to this new branch of science and to present evidence to dispel the old reefer madness myths that are used to continue law enforcement policies that derail, wreck and destroy the lives of otherwise decent people just because they use, grow or sell marijuana.

I hope that *Marijuana Gateway to Health* will inform the public that using marijuana or cannabis products can be very beneficial and explain why we have been so mistaken and mislead about its effects on the body. The first part of the book, "High Science," begins by explaining the endocannabinoid system—how it was discovered, how it operates and how the cannabinoids from marijuana interact with its receptors. The next chapters present the stunning evidence that cannabinoids, especially THC and CBD, interrupt a number of disease processes in a variety of surprising ways and therefore inhaling or ingesting marijuana benefits our health and vitality. The weight of the evidence is so great that no one who is considering the issue of marijuana prohibition from a scientific perspective can possibly justify the continuation of this destructive policy.

The second part of the book, "The Fall and Rise of Medical Marijuana" is a history of the medical marijuana movement, an examination of efforts to resuscitate reefer madness fears, a look at real concerns about problematic marijuana use and an overview of the state of the herb.

Ideally people will read this book, learn to talk about the data, begin conversations and work to eradicate the delusion that marijuana is a harmful substance of abuse that must be restricted by invading and brutalizing the lives of those who enjoy or need it. When we reach that point, we can really begin to work with the cannabis plant to create a healthier and happier world with fewer heartbreaking early deaths from cancer and neurological diseases.

PART ONE

HIGH SCIENCE

(1)

THE ENDOCANNABINOID SYSTEM

MARIJUANA HAS BEEN THE OBJECT of scorn and derision for nearly a century. Nicknamed "the evil weed," it has been the target of hysterical, multibillion dollar eradication campaigns intended to destroy the plant and eliminate its use. Yet it endures. Marijuana consumption is more popular than it has ever been. Drug warriors continue trying to persuade the public that marijuana is a dangerous substance, but their task is getting increasingly difficult as science uncovers more data about how marijuana really affects the body. After decades of unsupported fear-mongering, careful scientific research is now showing that marijuana is actually very good for our health. We now know that marijuana is not a gateway to drug addiction or illness. What the latest research makes clear is that, if marijuana is a gateway to anything, it is a gateway to health.

Marijuana is beginning to emerge from under a cloud of contempt because it has been at the center of one of the most exciting and underappreciated developments in biological science in recent times. Research on its psychological effects led directly to the discovery of a new chemical signaling system in the human body which is now recognized as playing a crucial role in regulating our neurology and physiology. It is becoming increasingly clear that this biological communication and regulatory system also powerfully affects the development and progression of numerous illnesses, especially cancer and Alzheimer's disease. In the context of the last hundred years of propaganda and prohibition, it is both ironic and amusing that this system never would have been discovered had it not been for the widespread "recreational" use of marijuana. The discovery of this profoundly important biological regulatory system—this new understanding of how our vital mental and physical functions work and remain in balance—arose from the search to find out how marijuana gets people high. Though the plant is commonly referred to as marijuana, it is also known by its Latin genus name, cannabis (this book will use the terms interchangeably). *Cannabinoids* are the unique chemical compounds found in marijuana, the most psychoactive and most studied of which is delta-9-tetrahydrocannabinol, or THC. As we will see, many of these compounds appear to have therapeutic applications. *Endocannabinoids* (endogenous cannabinoids) are mol-

> *Cannabis is the single most versatile herbal remedy on Earth. No other single plant contains as wide a range of medically active herbal constituents.*

ecules similar in structure and function to the cannabinoids produced by the cannabis plant, but they differ in that endocannabinoids are produced naturally within our bodies. These molecules act as the triggering and regulating agents for this physiological communications system, the *endocannabinoid system*, in the same way that serotonin or dopamine work in their own respective systems.

The endocannabinoid system is made up of the cannabinoids, cannabinoid (CB) receptors, as well as the chemical mechanisms responsible for synthesizing and eliminating both. Endocannabinoids are referred to as "endogenous ligands," molecules that turn certain biological activities on, off, up, and down, in part by binding to "receptor sites" on specific kinds of cells. Think of it in mechanical terms. Let's say you have a light switch with a dimmer, but there's no knob to adjust the dimmer so you're stuck in the dark. By pushing a knob onto the switch peg, you can turn on and adjust the brightness of the lights. Certain cannabinoids are like the knob—they fit the switch and provide a way to adjust its activity. Other cannabinoids regulate our health by influencing the biological activity of various systems, receptors and neurotransmitters. The endocannabinoid system does not act alone, it is a complex signaling network that influences numerous physiological pathways.

So what activities do cannabinoids help regulate? According to Dr. Raphael Mechoulam, one of the founding fathers of cannabinoid research, "There is barely a biological, physiological system in our bodies in which the endocannabinoids do not participate."[1] Decades of research have now shown that cannabinoids and endocannabinoids help regulate sleep, appetite, psychological well-being, and many more vital functions. They also help reduce the likelihood of certain kinds of diseases—including, as we will see, protecting the brain from Alzheimer's disease and suppressing and preventing cancer growth.

It is not an overstatement to refer to Dr. Raphael Mechoulam as a founding father of cannabinoid research. It was Mechoulam and his partner Dr. Yehiel Gaoni who first identified and synthesized THC, the principal psychoactive component of cannabis, while working at Hebrew University in Jerusalem in 1964. When Mechoulam began his career as a biochemical researcher in the early 1960s, he targeted cannabis as a field of investigation because "it was almost totally neglected," and "the active constituent(s) of cannabis had never been isolated in pure form and no definitive structure(s) had been put forth."[2]

Up to this point, the search for the agent responsible for the psychoactive effects of cannabis had been difficult. THC is just one member of a large family of similarly-constructed compounds, and it was difficult to tease them apart with the techniques then available to biochemists. It was not until the 1960s that technological advances such as chromatography and nuclear magnetic resonance enabled Mechoulam and his colleagues to isolate specific cannabinoids and determine how they differed from one another.

Mechoulam initiated his investigation into cannabis with "5 kg of superb, smuggled Lebanese hashish" provided by a friend at Police Headquarters.[3] The first research that Mechoulam undertook was to examine cannabidiol (CBD), a constituent of marijuana which had been chemically isolated from other cannabinoids but its chemical structure had not yet been defined. Using nuclear magnetic resonance (NMR; a technique that identifies molecular structures) as their primary tool, Mechoulam and colleague Yuval Shvo deciphered the molecular configuration of CBD. Like alchemists in search of the philosopher's stone, they began to dig deeper. As they searched for the elusive chemicals that produce the effects of the marijuana high the team tested molecule after molecule on rhesus monkeys until they finally identified a single psychoactive agent. Mechoulam later recalled that his team was very surprised that "only delta-9-THC affected the rhesus monkeys."[4]

Following this key discovery, Mechoulam continued to explore the nature and activity of cannabinoids. Interest in the field began to expand. Over the next 15 years, Mechoulam's group at Hebrew University and many other scientists in the United States, Europe, and Japan conducted a great deal of work on cannabinoids. Mechoulam recounted that during that time much was learned about the pharmacology, biochemistry, and medicinal effects of cannabinoids, yet their mode of action—how they did what they did—was still "an enigma."

Nearly a quarter century after Mechoulam's discovery of THC, Allyn Howlett, Ph.D., and her graduate student William Devane provided one of the first answers to the riddle of how cannabinoids work in the brain. In 1988, Howlett and Devane marked a synthetic cannabinoid with radioactive tritium in order to follow its path through a rat brain. In doing so, they were able to identify where the drug was binding in the brain. These docking sites were the first cannabinoid receptors to be identified. Howlett and her team published a paper announcing their discovery, affirming that a pharmacologically-distinct cannabinoid receptor had been located in brain tissue. This profound discovery led to the charting of a novel neurotransmitter system and the emergence of an entirely new branch of biological science. These receptor sites were designated CB1 (cannabinoid receptor number 1).

Howlett's discovery wasn't just a breakthrough for researchers interested in cannabis and cannabinoids—it also said something about the nature of biological signaling systems in general. "Receptors are not built into our brains or anywhere in our bodies because there is a plant out there that will produce a compound that acts on them, that just doesn't work that way," Raphael Mechoulam later explained. "Receptors are found in our bodies because we produce compounds that act upon those receptors."[5] In the wake of Howlett's discovery, scientists intensified their search for the endogenous cannabinoids that they knew would match the newly discovered CB1 receptor sites.

In 1992 Czech chemist Lumír Ondřej Hanuš and William Devane were working at Mechoulam's lab at Hebrew University when they identified an endogenous compound that fit the CB1 receptor like a key in a lock. They named this new endocannabinoid anandamide after the Sanskrit word *ananda*—"ecstasy" or "supreme bliss." The discovery of anandamide was trumpeted in the media with sensational headlines about "the body's own marijuana" and stories that tended to discount the profundity of the discovery with a dismissive air of stoner whimsy.

Nevertheless marijuana and cannabinoid research was gaining respect among a growing number of clinical investigators. In 1993, a research group at Cambridge University's Medical Research Council led by Sean Munro, Ph.D., identified and successfully cloned the second cannabinoid receptor, CB2. Two years later, in 1995, Mechoulam made another historic discovery when he isolated a second endocannabinoid, 2-arachidonoylglycerol (2AG) from spleen tissue. Other scientists began plotting the distribution (or "expression") of the corresponding receptors throughout the body and soon uncovered the surprising extent of the endocannabinoid system's regulatory functions.

It is now increasingly recognized that the discovery of the existence and scale of the endocannabinoid system represents a significant advancement in our understanding of human biology. According to Professor Leslie Iversen of the Department of Pharmacology at the University of Oxford in the U.K., "These discoveries shed entirely new light on the pharmacology of cannabis. From the original goal of studying a psychotropic plant cannabinoid, we now see instead the opportunity of revealing a wholly novel physiological control system in the body."[6] As author Michael Pollan writes in his immensely popular and influential book *The Botany of Desire,* "Someday soon Mechoulam and Howlett will almost surely receive the Nobel Prize, for their discoveries opened a new branch of neuroscience that promises to revolutionize our understanding of the brain and lead to a whole new class of drugs."[7]

Cannabinoid and cannabinoid receptor research is still in an early phase but, as Pollan points out, a revolution is underway. This new branch of biological science is still in its embryonic stage and important revelations lay ahead, such as the possible discovery of other endocannabinoids and their receptors, how they influence the regulation of various body systems, and how they may themselves be affected by other cannabinoids and cannabis compounds such as terpenes (which are responsible for the distinct odor of cannabis and its preparations). Although this field of research has been limited to a small number of labs worldwide, scientists already have a fairly strong grasp of how cannabinoid receptors and endocannabinoids function and what they regulate. Cannabinoid receptors belong to a class of biological structures known as G protein-coupled receptors (GPCRs) which relay signals through the cell membrane into the cell in order to influence its activity. Cannabinoids activate specific kinds of these receptors to convert extracellular stimuli into intracellular signals.

Endocannabinoids are not the only compounds that act on the endocannabinoid system. Cannabinoids found outside the body are known as exocannabinoids, and these include the naturally-occurring chemicals we have already discussed such as THC and CBD. Cannabinoids found in the marijuana plant are also known as phytocannabinoids. Scientists are also producing synthetic cannabinoids with names like WIN-55212-2. Cannabinoids work by bonding to the cannabinoid receptors in the body, which then send signals into cells that alter their activity. The CB1 receptor is most abundantly expressed in the central nervous system (CNS), but it is also found in many other parts of the body. CB1 receptors are also concentrated in adipose tissue (fat) as well as the stomach, placenta, lungs, uterus, and liver.

CB2 receptors are also widespread, existing in the liver, spleen, gastrointestinal tract, heart, kidney, bones, endocrine glands, lymph and immune cells, and the peripheral nervous system. Although the scope of their activity is only beginning to be appreciated, it is clear that CB2 receptors are involved with everything from digestion to bone strength to the perception of pain. Claims of marijuana's broad therapeutic effectiveness were easier to dismiss before we learned about the wide distribution of cannabinoid receptors in the body. Now, those claims are starting to make a lot more sense.

The wide distribution of cannabinoid receptors explains why they can have such powerful effects on appetite, blood pressure, cerebral blood flow, digestion, nausea, immune function, memory, mood, movement, neurological health, pain, reproduction, stress response and more. It seems that everywhere in the body cannabinoid receptors are regulating activity and maintaining health. The sheer ubiquity of the endocannabinoid system and the immense diversity of cannabinoids that exist both inside and outside the body has convinced many experts of marijuana's medical potential. One of these experts, Dr. Ethan Russo, has said, "Cannabis is the single most versatile herbal remedy on Earth. No other single plant contains as wide a range of medically active herbal constituents."[8]

Science has completely altered our understanding of marijuana. It no longer makes sense to criminalize marijuana users and demonize the plant as a toxic menace or the devil's weed. The new scientific reality is in fact just the opposite: marijuana is a natural ally of the human body, capable of interacting with any number of body systems to protect us from a variety of terrible, degenerative diseases. Given the extensive influence of cannabinoids in the body, it should not surprise us that marijuana has numerous beneficial effects. But what are those beneficial effects, and how might they be maximized?

Ⓒ

SMOKING OUT LUNG CANCER

THOUGH IT MAY BE HARD to believe at first, there is a large and growing body of evidence that smoking marijuana reduces your chances of getting lung cancer. Given what we know about the role that smoking tobacco plays in the development of lung cancer, it seems counterintuitive and even ironic that smoking anything could work against the disease. Nevertheless, it appears that chronic, long-term marijuana smokers actually have lower rates of lung cancer than nonsmokers. We are constantly learning more about how the cannabinoids found in marijuana protect us from cancer in a variety of ways.

The first real evidence of marijuana's anti-carcinogenic properties appeared back in 1975, when the remarkable and somewhat shocking results of an oncology research project were published in the respected Journal of the National Cancer Institute. In the paper, "Anticancer Activity of Cannabinoids," researchers at Virginia Commonwealth University described how the growth of a certain type of lung cancer in mice was inhibited by the oral administration of three naturally-occurring cannabinoids—delta-9-tetrahydrocannabinol (delta-9-THC), delta-8-tetrahydrocannabinol (delta-8-THC), and cannabinol (CBN).[9] The scientists also discovered that the degree to which tumors were prevented from growing depended on the amount of cannabinoids administered, and that delta-9-THC also seemed to effectively reduce spleen inflammation associated with leukemia. Furthermore, they found that bone marrow treated with delta-8-THC and delta-9-THC showed a dose-dependent resistance to cancer.[10]

Although these surprising results were reported in The Washington Post, they were unfortunately treated as an anomaly rather than as a promising new field of research. The findings were inconvenient for the new "War on Drugs" that President Nixon had launched with great enthusiasm just five years earlier. Shortly after this study was published, Congress established the National Institute on Drug Abuse (NIDA) to be the national gatekeeper of all research into illegal drugs and substances, and gave it a strict mandate to research only the harm posed by such compounds. Any research into the possible benefits of marijuana or cannabinoids was subsequently forbidden, and the study was ignored.

It took over two decades for the next U.S.-based research indicating that cannabis has powerful anti-carcinogenic properties to emerge. In 1996, AIDS specialist Donald Abrams, M.D., became aware of a study revealing the beneficial effects of cannabinoids that was being buried by government officials. Abrams, whose battle with NIDA for the right to conduct research into marijuana's benefits for AIDS patients had put him in the public eye, received a document from an investigative journalist describing the results of a government-funded study of the possible carcinogenic effects of cannabinoids. The study was intended to determine the toxicity of THC in rats and mice and to find out how likely it was to induce cancer.

In a cover letter, the reporter told Abrams that the paper was a draft version with limited distribution, and that government officials were attempting to prevent the public release of the final version. In most cases, such documents are made available within six months of the publication of the draft. Yet in this case, two full years had passed and the final version still had not appeared—despite the legal requirement that all research funded by tax dollars be made publicly available. When he received the report, Abrams was in the midst of an intense battle with the federal government over its prevention of research into the possible benefits of marijuana. He was immediately suspicious as to why the final version of the report was still missing in action two years later—and his suspicion grew when he read the study's conclusions.

Abrams called the principal investigator of the National Toxicology Project, the group that had conducted the study. The researcher was astounded that the final report had not been released and wondered if the data was being actively suppressed. When he contacted the authorities who were supposed to be responsible for releasing the study, he was told that the delay had been "just an oversight" and that the final version would be released immediately. It is peculiar how selective these government "oversights" can be.

So what were the bureaucrats trying to conceal? Contrary to the government's hopes, rats and mice which were orally dosed with varying levels of pure THC had a significantly greater survival rate than those that were not.[11] It was discovered that THC was effective in reducing cancer of the breast, uterus, pancreas, and testicles and that higher doses led to greater protection and longer life. It was hardly surprising that federal health and anti-drug agencies, who only wanted to know about the damaging effects of marijuana, did not want such results released to the public.

> *It was discovered that THC was effective in reducing cancer of the breast, uterus, pancreas, and testes and that higher doses led to greater protection and longer life.*

One can only wonder how many other studies have not seen the light of day because of inconvenient results, and have disappeared down the Orwellian memory hole.

But now we know the wonderful and startling truth. According to this and other studies, if you ingest marijuana's psychoactive cannabinoid, THC, you just might live longer. Marijuana is apparently very good for you—like blueberries or broccoli.

More evidence that marijuana works against lung cancer came in 2006 from a NIDA-funded study that was intended to prove once and for all that long-term marijuana smoking causes lung cancer. Pulmonologist Donald Tashkin, M.D. is NIDA's go-to-guy on the effects of marijuana on lung function. When he began the study, he was certain that there was a positive link between chronic marijuana use and lung cancer. "Marijuana smoke contains a similar profile for carcinogens in tobacco smoke," explained Tashkin in a public interview. "It's not an unreasonable hypothesis that marijuana would also cause lung cancer."[12]

Tashkin and his team at the University of California, Los Angeles fully expected that by conducting a carefully-designed, epidemiological study they would settle the question and finally prove that smoking marijuana increases the incidence of lung cancer in long-term users. The researchers examined more than 1200 cases of lung, head and neck, and esophageal cancer patients and compared them to more than 1000 healthy control subjects. Their work was overseen by one of the world's top experts on case-controlled methodology.

After the data was processed and adjusted for factors such as alcohol or cigarette use, age, and family history, the scientists were amazed (and some were appalled). According to the data, marijuana did not cause lung cancer. Not only that, but the data suggested that it actually inhibited the formation and growth of cancer cells. The study had shown that marijuana had a "protective effect," preventing or reducing the risk of tumors.[13] According to the study, chronic, long-term smokers of marijuana reduced their likelihood of developing lung cancer by as much as 37 percent when compared with nonsmokers.

For the first time, a major epidemiological study confirmed the clinical data on the role of cannabinoid receptors in suppressing cancer. It provided solid evidence that marijuana smokers are less likely to develop lung cancer than nonsmokers. Tashkin had to admit that his team had "failed to find any positive association between marijuana use [and cancer], even heavy marijuana use. If anything the risks were a little bit less."[14]

Six months later, in April 2007, a group of Harvard scientists shared the results of their own research. Their results seemed to confirm Tashkin's research and suggested some possible mechanisms by which marijuana achieved its cancer-fighting effects. Anju Preet, Ph.D., the lead researcher for the Harvard study, told the American Association for Cancer Prevention that when mice with lung cancer were given THC their tumors were reduced by half and the spread of the disease was slowed. Preet suggested on the basis of the results that THC's therapeutic effects may have something to do with its direct effect on cancer cells. She explained, "THC can have a potential therapeutic role. Maybe THC is killing cells. The preliminary studies are promising."[15] Specifically, Preet's study showed that tumor cells treated with THC had reductions in *epidermal growth factor receptors,* or EGFR, which is found in high levels in aggressive and treatment-resistant tumors. Along with shrinking tumors to half their original size, THC was associated with a 60 percent reduction in cancer lesions in the lungs of the mice. Preet went on to suggest that because lung cancer cells have a similar biochemistry involving the expression of EGFR as tumors of the head, neck, colon, and pancreas, these other types of cancer might also respond positively to treatment with THC or marijuana.

Unfortunately, despite clear evidence from solid scientific studies, many people—including some researchers themselves—still find it hard to believe that marijuana use can improve our health. In the abstract for the UCLA study conducted by Tashkin and colleagues, the researchers were so incredulous of their results that they questioned the validity of their own data. When it comes to marijuana research, it seems that far too many scientists have a hard time admitting confidence in their unexpected results. In the first line of the conclusions section of the abstract, the authors wrote, "Our results may have been affected by selection bias or error in measuring lifetime exposure and confounder histories; but they suggest that the association of these cancers with marijuana, even long-term or heavy use, is not strong and may be below practically detectable limits."[16]

What the researchers seemed to be saying was that they could not believe what their research revealed, despite the fact that it used state-of-the-art methodology and was overseen by the world's top expert in the field. Instead, they thought that they must have made some mistake because it was inconceivable that marijuana could fight cancer. Perhaps they were afraid (with good reason) that if their research did show a positive link between THC and tumor reduction, they would never get funding for that type of research again. Based on NIDA's goals for funding marijuana studies, it is reasonable to assume that different results would have led the scientists to present their conclusions in a very different way. Their conclusion simply did not acknowledge the study's most important result—that THC had a protective effect against lung cancer—relegating it to the status of an interesting, though unimportant, side observation. However careful and thorough the research might have been, their conclusions were mired in politics.

Despite the early intrusion of politics into the study's findings, it should be noted that the lead researcher has subsequently been very forthcoming with the positive results. After more than 30 years of cooperating with NIDA to try to prove that marijuana is harmful, Tashkin has recently endorsed legalization. "Early on, when our research appeared as if there would be a negative impact on lung health, I was opposed to legalization because I thought it would lead to increased use and that would lead to increased health effects," he recently explained. "But at this point, I'd be in favor of legalization."[17] The mark of a true and honest scientist is the ability to change one's views when presented with substantial evidence to the contrary. Though he began with some strong biases against marijuana, he changed his position when the science contradicted his preconceived notions.

As one of the few herbal substances proven to have cancer-fighting properties, cannabis is a drug warrior's nightmare. For many years, prohibition, politics and bias hobbled any efforts to understand marijuana's therapeutic applications. Fortunately, as more studies are published revealing cannabis' anticancer activity, a growing number of international medical experts are abandoning the prejudicial notion that the plant and its constituents are dangerous with no redeeming qualities and they are beginning to conduct untainted research. Many of these new studies are uncovering unexpected health benefits of cannabinoids that even extend beyond cancer protection.

Knowledge that the endocannabinoid system is involved in many of these positive effects has given researchers a path to follow in their investigations of marijuana's contributions to health and well-being. As the field of cannabis research expands, we can expect more startling results about how smoking or ingesting marijuana can improve human health by fighting disease and—just as importantly—enhancing mood.

③

FIGHTING OTHER CANCERS

CANCER—THE VERY WORD CARRIES WITH it a powerful sense of dread and fear. It can appear suddenly with little or no warning, rapidly diminishing, disfiguring, and destroying life. There is almost certainly no other disease in developed nations that causes as much depression and grief as does cancer. As advances in medicine and public health bring other causes of premature mortality under control, cancer moves to the forefront as the preeminent killer. The marketing of supplements to prevent cancer is a multibillion dollar industry, primarily a multibillion dollar snake-oil industry. But suddenly we find a substance from a plant that really does work against a number of cancers, and ironically it's illegal because it's supposed to be harmful.

The term cancer refers to any of a number of various manifestations of abnormal cell growth, so when we say that marijuana fights cancer it is important to be clear what kind of cancer we are referring to. But first, what is cancer?

Simply put, cancer is cell reproduction gone awry. It begins when healthy, working cells mutate into irregular cells that do not function appropriately and divide more rapidly. How and why this mutation happens varies between cancers and cell types. In all cases, however, the mutated cells get stuck in an immature reproductive state and fail to assume their proper functions. These mutated cells then generate even more dysfunctional cells, and as they grow they crowd out and impede the work of surrounding functional cells. The growing clumps of abnormal cells ultimately form a mass called a malignancy or tumor, the presence of which wreaks havoc on bodily structures, activities, and metabolism. Cancer is like a body snatcher that arises from within, stealing away organ function, nutrients, and (all too often) life itself. As Sherwin Nuland wrote in his book *How We Die,* cancer "pursues a continuous, uninhibited, circumferential, barn-burning expedition of destructiveness, in which it heeds no rules, follows no commands, [and] explodes all resistance in a homicidal riot of destructiveness."[18]

> *Cannabinoids may be an effective therapeutic option for treating highly invasive cancers.*

As they grow, tumors induce a variety of alterations and abnormalities in the way the body utilizes carbohydrates, fats, and proteins. Some even release the substance cachectin, which suppresses appetite by chemically altering the function of the brain's feeding center. This is what induces the shocking emaciation so often associated with cancer. In these cases, it becomes difficult for a patient to ingest enough nutrients to nourish the body and also feed the voracious tumor because the tumor is suppressing the desire to eat. The resulting malnourishment in turn weakens resistance to other diseases. Tumors also release substances which suppress the immune system, making infections one of the leading causes of death in cancer patients.

Some tumors are located in non-vital organs and structures (like the breast or prostate) and would not be life-threatening were it not for their tendency to spread to other areas. Eventually, they overtake and compromise the walls of blood or lymph vessels. At this point, the tumor comes into direct contact with blood or lymph (the fluid found between the cells of the body), and uses these streams to colonize other tissues or organs such as the bones, lungs, or liver in a process called metastasis. New tumors then grow at these sites, shedding additional cells into even more areas until the body is riddled with abnormal growths. It is then often only a matter of time until one of these growths deals the final mortal blow.

If, as so much research indicates, cannabis suppresses cancer, how does it do this? Although no one knows for certain, it could be the result of a variety of actions. According to cannabis researchers Donald Abrams, M.D., and Manuel Guzman, Ph.D., cannabinoids seem to work against cancer through a number of different mechanisms including killing mutated cells, slowing their growth, or preventing them from spreading or growing new blood vessels.[19] In fact, there is evidence that the cannabinoids found in marijuana have the ability to identify mutated cells, stunt their growth, cut off their blood supply, and prevent them from spreading before they can get a foothold and form tumors.

Could cannabis be a wonder drug? We have been so brainwashed to think in negative (and even criminal) terms about marijuana that it is hard for some people to open their minds to the possibility that marijuana is a beneficial and even life-preserving substance. But as we learn more and more about marijuana, it is becoming quite clear that it is helpful rather than harmful. This is not some wacky pipe dream that the Fabulous Furry Freak Brothers had after eating too many hash brownies; it is supported by solid, peer-reviewed clinical and epidemiological scientific data from around the world.

One way that cannabinoids kill cancer cells is through a process known as cell apoptosis, or programmed cell death. Apoptosis is a Greek term, meaning the falling away of leaves, that is currently used to describe the natural death progression of cells. One of the problems with cancer cells is that they do not follow the normal life and death cycle of other cells. Instead of dying naturally they continue growing, crowding out and starving the surrounding healthy cells. There is evidence that cannabinoids selectively trigger the death of unruly cancer cells before they are able to spread and encroach on other cells while leaving healthy cells alone.

A 2006 study conducted by a group of Spanish researchers, for example, found that cannabinoids induced apoptosis and reduced tumor growth in animal models of pancreatic cancer, preventing the spread of pancreatic tumor cells.[20] The pancreas is an organ situated below the stomach, and is involved in producing certain hormones and digestive enzymes. Unfortunately, by the time cancer is discovered in the pancreas, it has often metastasized to the nearby liver. As a result, death from pancreatic cancer is grueling and painful and usually occurs less than two years after diagnosis. About 35,000 people die of pancreatic cancer each year in the U.S.

Research from Italy also supports the data concerning cannabis' anti-tumor activity. In 2008, another group of researchers discovered that the activation of cannabinoid receptors CB1 and CB2 produces apoptosis in colon cancer cells.[21] Colon cancer is the second leading cause of cancer-related deaths in the United States. If marijuana turns out to be as effective against cancer as this data suggests, then health authorities may find it useful to issue guidelines for effective marijuana use to those with a family history of the illness.

Marijuana also has powerful anti-inflammatory properties that may work to keep healthy cells from turning malignant in the first place. Inflammation from either infection or irritation can increase the likelihood of cancer by continuously stimulating the pathways that control cellular growth and division, DNA repair, and other physiological processes. The cannabinoids found in marijuana work against this inflammation. This anti-inflammatory action is also apparently what makes cannabis effective against arthritis and a number of other pain syndromes.

THC also works against other cancers by acting as a powerful antiviral agent, inhibiting the spread of at least one type of cancer-causing virus. Scientists at the University of South Florida found that THC "specifically targets the viral and/or cellular mechanisms required for replication" and prevents the replication of certain kinds of herpes viruses.[22] The Florida study only investigated the gamma herpesvirus, not the herpes simplex virus associated with cold sores and genital herpes. THC's effectiveness against the gamma herpesvirus is important because it is implicated in the development of many malignancies, including Hodgkin's disease, Kaposi's sarcoma, Epstein-Barr virus, Burkitt's lymphoma, nasopharyngeal carcinoma, and AIDS-associated lymphoma.

Biology and medical text books will have to be rewritten to explain that there is solid scientific evidence that cannabis helps the body to ward off the growth and spread of cancers of the lung, pancreas, and colon—and that this same action seems to work to keep other forms of cancer suppressed. Research conducted in Germany demonstrating that cannabinoids inhibit the spread of cervical cancer cells has led scientists to conclude that cannabinoids may be an effective therapeutic option for treating highly invasive cancers.[23] The very title of the study is encouraging: "Inhibition of Cancer Cell Invasion by Cannabinoids."

These studies are not flukes. What we see when looking at the science of cannabis and cannabinoids is a consistent pattern of protection from cancer and other diseases. As more studies are conducted on cannabis' effectiveness against cancer, we are likely to find even more types of tumors that it works against. But even now, at the dawn of the renaissance of medical cannabis research, study after study indicates that it is a plant loaded with beneficial compounds that can help us to maintain optimum health. What else does the hard science have to say?

Research from Sweden has recently found that endogenous and some synthetic cannabinoids help prevent various kinds of cancer and lymphoma from spreading out of control.[24] Specifically, it appears that activating cannabinoid receptors with cannabinoids helps to inhibit the growth of certain kinds of lymphoma. A 1999 study from the University of California, San Francisco supported these findings, linking continuing marijuana use among men to a decreased risk of non-Hodgkin's lymphoma.[25] There is also evidence that cannabinoids prevent the formation of blood vessels by tumors, a process known as angiogenesis.[26] Angiogenesis refers to the growing of new blood vessels, and although it is necessary for the survival of healthy cells it is also how tumors deprive surrounding healthy tissues of nourishment.

In another study from Spain, Manuel Guzman, Ph.D. and colleagues have shown that cannabinoids "induced a considerable growth inhibition of malignant tumors," by triggering the cancer cells to die off and by blocking angiogenesis in certain skin cancers.[27]

Guzman and his team have also made some remarkable discoveries concerning the effects of cannabinoids—especially delta-9-THC—on suppressing the growth of glioblastoma, the most devastating form of brain cancer. While studying fat oxidation in the brain and the effect of various drugs on brain metabolism, Guzman and his colleagues "found some surprising actions that prompted [them] to study more in detail the molecular bases of how cannabinoids act on brain cells." Guzman explained that "On one hand, we were interested in the possibility that cannabinoids protected some types of brain cells from toxic compounds and situations. On the other hand we conducted some experiments with brain cancer cells and found that cannabinoids killed them."[28]

They found that cannabinoids effectively impaired the function of vascular endothelial growth factor (VEGF), which is necessary for a tumor to establish a blood supply via angiogenesis. Without the ability to create blood vessels to bring nourishment, the tumor cannot grow.

The research data indicating that cannabinoids apparently target and destroy the brain cancer cells, while sparing the surrounding healthy cells and perhaps even protecting them, is even more astonishing. Guzman's team found that although cannabinoids destroy tumor cells, they leave their healthy counterparts intact and may even have a protective function.[29] Perhaps the biggest problem with traditional chemotherapy is that it does not distinguish between tumor cells and healthy cells, which results in nausea, anemia and hair loss as gut and hair cells are wiped out along with cancer cells. These studies seem to suggest that cannabinoid compounds could be developed to be used as safe and effective chemotherapy agents.

Cannabinoids induced a considerable growth inhibition of malignant tumors, by triggering the cancer cells to die off and by blocking angiogenesis in certain skin cancers.

These researchers also found that cannabinoids prevent the growth of and encourage the death of certain prostate cancer cells and reduce tumor growth in mice.[30] Isn't it thrilling to know that cannabinoids stunt and starve tumor cells? The research conducted by Guzman and others on cannabinoids has inspired a growing number of investigators to study the possible uses of these unfairly demonized compounds against other cancers.

Another interesting study found that although THC's ability to kill prostate cancer cells depended on the amount of THC administered, it surprisingly had nothing to do with THC's action on cannabinoid receptors.[31] This indicates that THC fights tumors by inducing their deaths in more than one way. When THC's effect on the cannabinoid receptors was blocked, it still caused the tumor to wither and die. This is remarkable; it means that marijuana makes one's body hostile to cancer both by activating the cannabinoid receptors and by exposing cells directly to THC.

A group of Thai scientists found that THC worked similarly against bile duct cancer (cholangiocarcinoma) by preventing tumor cells from reproducing, migrating, and invading other areas as well as by causing apoptosis. The effects were so profound that the researchers proposed that THC be used as a regular treatment for cholangiocarcinoma, which is devastating and difficult to treat.[32]

Promising research from Guzman and his team has also showed that THC prevents aggressive breast cancers from proliferating and generating blood vessels, and increases their rate of death.[33] Experiments conducted with the non-psychoactive cannabinoid CBD have also shown promising results for preventing the spread of breast cancer. Breast cancer takes about 40,000 lives in the U.S. annually. Reducing those numbers by using cannabinoids would alleviate a lot of heartbreak and grief. Research will undoubtedly continue to uncover more about how marijuana works to keep bodies safe and healthy.

Researchers at Upstate Medical University in Syracuse, New York, looked at the effects of cannabinoids at the cellular level to try to understand how they might be exerting their anti-cancer effects. In their study, they found that both delta-9-THC and delta-8-THC caused a sharp decline in the respiratory rate of oral cancer cells.[34] The effects were directly related to the concentration of THC on and around the cancer cells, and delta-9-THC was the more potent of the two compounds tested.[35] Also interesting is the fact that the endocannabinoid anandamide did not effectively block the cancer cells' respiration, which indicates that the effects of delta-8-THC and delta-9-THC were not mediated by cannabinoid receptors.[36] It is stunning that the cannabinoids in marijuana have such multifaceted activity against cancer cells. Not only do THC and other phytocannabinoids trigger the cannabinoid receptors to suppress and kill cancer cells, but they also directly target unruly cells for death by suffocation and other methods.

For more evidence that that marijuana use can be part of a healthy, cancer-resistant lifestyle, consider the results of another study. This one, conducted by a wide range of collaborators from several respected academic institutions, found that individuals who had used marijuana for 10 to 20 years had a significantly reduced risk of carcinoma of the head and neck.[37] Here we have even more epidemiological data that supports the clinical findings that marijuana has anticancer properties. These results are simply amazing. Just as with lung cancer, we can see that regular, long-term marijuana use may be powerfully protective against developing other kinds of cancer. By contrast, the regular use of alcohol—a legal drug—is associated with a significantly increased risk of these same diseases.

This is the current state of knowledge about marijuana's anti-cancer properties. Extensive clinical studies reveal that the cannabinoids found in marijuana act in a number of ways to suppress the survival, growth, and spread of a wide variety of cancer cells. The activation of cannabinoid receptors generates compounds and actions that are hostile to cancer, but cannabinoids also act independently of the receptors, biochemically nourishing healthy cells while attacking unhealthy ones. Epidemiological population studies confirm these findings with evidence that regular marijuana users are less likely to develop certain cancers than are nonsmokers.

$$\textcircled{4}$$

ALZHEIMER'S AND DEMENTIA: HOW CANNABIS HELPS

IT IS A TOUGH CALL, whether cancer or Alzheimer's disease is the more dreaded illness. The creeping loss of mind and self that is Alzheimer's dementia, a kind of confused and suspended animation, is a terrifying and debilitating experience for both patient and family. Thankfully, one of the most effective things one can do to prevent it is to smoke or eat marijuana, which protects us from Alzheimer's and other forms of dementia by stimulating the brain to generate new brain cells, or neurons, and by reducing neuroinflammation. It is another tough call, whether it is more surprising that marijuana works against lung cancer or that it protects the brain from Alzheimer's disease.

The human brain is made up of about 100 billion neurons which communicate through vast neural networks. Alzheimer's disease is a progressive and fatal brain disease that destroys those pathways of communication by generating deposits (or plaques) and tangles on and around neurons, destroying the pathways and preventing neurons from properly communicating. These plaques and tangles were first described in the medical literature in 1906 by Dr. Alois Alzheimer, who found them in the brain of a demented patient while performing surgery. We now know that the plaques are made of amyloid beta, a protein fragment that builds up between the nerve cells. The tangles of nerve fibers described by Alzheimer, by contrast, build up inside dying cells. The exact mechanism by which these aberrations cause the dementia typical of Alzheimer's disease is as yet unknown. What is known is that THC, the principal psychoactive component of marijuana, can help to prevent them from occurring. In 2006, researchers at the world-renowned Scripps Institute in La Jolla, California announced that THC is more effective at preventing Alzheimer's disease than any other substance or drug.

Kim Janda, the spokesperson for the study, stated that while the researchers were "certainly not advocating the use of illegal drugs, these findings offer convincing evidence that THC possesses remarkable inhibitory qualities," especially when compared to currently available treatments. Acetylcholinesterase (AChE) is an enzyme found naturally in the human body that contributes to the formation of the amyloid beta (AB) plaques common to Alzheimer's, and drugs

Cannabidiol, protected brain cells to a greater degree than either the dietary antioxidants vitamin E or vitamin C.

that block its action are known as AChE inhibitors. These chemicals are standard treatments for Alzheimer's, but the Scripps study found that "THC is a considerably superior inhibitor of AB aggregation" than AChE inhibitors and "may directly impact the progression of this debilitating disease."[38] The way that THC works to prevent the progression of Alzheimer's disease, Janda added, is a "previously unrecognized molecular mechanism" and an important breakthrough for medical science.[39]

Let's look at this in more detail. The plaques and tangles in the brain associated with Alzheimer's disease disrupt the signals between neurons. This causes mental function to deteriorate until the perception of time, the performance of routines, and the recollection of basic knowledge become difficult or impossible—this is the dementia that characterizes the disease. As the disease progresses, memories vanish and patients lose reference points for their lives. They fail to recognize friends and loved ones, and cherished memories and interests dissolve away until there is little left but a frightened and confused shell of a human. During this progressive dissolution, patients sometimes become angry and violent toward those who are closest to them, seeing them as threatening intruders. The degeneration progresses steadily, and although the rate at which it occurs varies from patient to patient, they all end up lost in a meaningless world. At this point, families often have no choice but to institutionalize their suffering loved one—which can be horribly expensive, especially considering that the body can live for a long time after the mind is gone. The greatest tragedy may be that Alzheimer's primarily affects only the areas of the brain involved in cognition, and not those involved with vital functions. It would be far more humane for both patients and their families if the body died along with the mind. Instead, death by Alzheimer's disease usually results from some type of infection. As the mind dies and patients enter a vegetative state, they forget vital skills such as how to urinate, defecate, chew, and swallow. Lying in their own waste, with decreased blood flow patients frequently develop skin infections which become growing, pus-filled bedsores that pour toxins into the bloodstream. Some patients choke to death on their own saliva or die of pneumonia from inhaling smaller amounts of it.

If marijuana can prevent or minimize this disease process, why aren't we being told about it? Is marijuana's euphoric effect so dangerous that we should reject its use and risk dying in pools of our own filth with ulcerating sores as we thrash against restraints, unaware of who we are? This aversion to using marijuana is "euphoranoia"—the irrational fear of getting high. There is no justification for keeping the public in the dark about marijuana's medical value when there are so many legal drugs that are much more dangerous to both our physical and mental health.

Alzheimer's is such a degrading descent into misery that one would expect our government to acknowledge the research and begin working to make marijuana-based medicines available to those at risk of developing dementia. Statistics show that with the aging baby boomer generation, 7.7 million people are expected to be diagnosed with Alzheimer's disease by the year 2030. This number could grow to 16 million by the year 2050 if something is not done to prevent it. The cost of care and the enormity of suffering associated with these numbers are horrifying to consider.

An urgent move to develop cannabis therapies for Alzheimer's patients should be underway, especially because of the complete lack of effective conventional treatments. A report in an online medical journal recently asked, "Is There Hope for [a] Novel Alzheimer's Agent?" Dimebon, a promising new drug intended to treat Alzheimer's disease, proved to be "a major disappointment" because it showed "absolutely zero effect" in multinational Phase 3 clinical trials.[40]

Let's look at more evidence that cannabis is effective for preventing and treating Alzheimer's dementia. Shortly after the publication of the Scripps THC/Alzheimer's study, the findings of a clinical trial conducted at Ohio State University supported its conclusions. According to researcher Gary Wenk, a synthetic cannabinoid known as WIN-55212-2 "substantially improved the memories of... older rats."[41] These older rats, which were injected with an inflammatory drug that creates the symptoms of Alzheimer's, improved substantially after receiving treatment with the cannabinoid. Wenk noted that the study was probably "a pretty good indication of how humans would respond to this drug."

Like so many other researchers, Wenk was initially reluctant to advocate using cannabinoids for preventing disease. He argued that WIN-55212-2 "is not a candidate for use in humans because it still contains substances that could trigger a high."[42] He also explained that he did not want to use real marijuana in his experiments "because we're trying to find a compound that isn't psychoactive."[43] Evidently our culture's euphoranoia is so extensive that getting high is considered a greater threat than dying of cancer or Alzheimer's.

Although, when later asked if people could smoke marijuana to prevent Alzheimer's disease if it runs in their family, Wenk admitted, "We're not saying that but it might actually work."[44]

After conducting further research, Dr. Wenk began to openly discuss the possibility that using marijuana is beneficial for brain health. He wrote an article for *Psychology Today* in which he stated that smoking marijuana "may also protect against some aspects of age-associated memory loss" because "Research in my laboratory has demonstrated that stimulating the brain's marijuana receptors may offer protection by reducing brain inflammation and by restoring neurogenesis."[45]

A study from the Guzman research team in Madrid, which conducted much of the cannabis and cancer research discussed in previous chapters, produced similar findings regarding cannabis and Alzheimer's disease. They concluded that "cannabinoids succeed in preventing the neurodegenerative process occurring in the disease."[46]

An abstract in the British Journal of Pharmacology also reviewed the anti-Alzheimer's activity of cannabinoids and concluded that, "cannabinoids offer a multi-faceted approach for the treatment of Alzheimer's disease by providing neuroprotection and reducing neuroinflammation, whilst simultaneously supporting the brain's intrinsic repair mechanisms by augmenting neurotrophin [a protein that protects brain cells] expression and enhancing neurogenesis [the growth of new brain cells]."[47] It is incredibly exciting to learn that cannabinoids work against this horrible disease in not just one but several ways: by protecting the brain, by eradicating a primary cause of the disease, and by stimulating the formation of functional new brain cells.

According to cutting-edge research, ingesting cannabis is one of the best things you can do for the health of your brain. This is bad news for the ideologically-blinded prohibitionists, but the majority of current scientific data clearly demonstrates that using marijuana is good for your brain.

Chronic use of marijuana may actually improve learning memory.

Xia Zhang, Associate Professor with the Neuropsychiatry Research Unit at the University of Saskatoon, admitted that the results of his research on cannabinoids and brain function were "quite a surprise." He discovered that the chronic use of marijuana could actually improve learning and memory.[48] It does this by promoting the growth of neurons in the hippocampus, an area of the brain important for learning and memory. Research shows that "cannabinoids are the only illicit drug that can promote adult hippocampal neurogenesis following chronic administration."[49] This activity creates antidepressant-like effects. Marijuana is truly a unique substance. It helps the brain generate new brain cells while simultaneously protecting the older ones.

How is it that our beliefs about cannabis have been so wrong? Why has so much of the marijuana-naïve public believed that the plant is damaging to the brain when it actually protects and nourishes it? The reason is that for years our tax dollars have been spent on generating pseudoscience that has been used to promote the anti-marijuana agenda of those with vested interests in the War on Drugs. The misconception that marijuana harms the brain is a perfect example of the social damage that can be done when biased scientists and agenda-driven ideologues use science to promote their cause.

In his book *On Fact and Fraud: Cautionary Tales from the Front Lines of Science,* David Goldstein of Caltech defines research misconduct as "fabrication, falsification, or plagiarism in proposing, performing, or reviewing research, or in reporting research results" which are "committed intentionally, or knowingly, or in reckless disregard of accepted practices."[50] This is an apt description of the fraudulent reefer madness research that the U.S. government has been supporting for years.

Perhaps the most egregious of these efforts to use science to support ideology were the monkey suffocation studies conducted at Tulane University in the 1970s. Hoping to prove definitively that marijuana caused brain damage, Dr. Robert Heath of the Tulane School of Medicine implanted the brains of rhesus monkeys with electrodes before forcing them to inhale concentrated marijuana smoke nearly to the point of suffocation. After the monkeys were killed and examined, the researchers found signs of brain damage in those asphyxiated with marijuana smoke but not in those who were allowed to breathe normally. Ronald Reagan cited this research as a reason to stop then-ongoing efforts for marijuana decriminalization and escalate the War on Drugs. The Tulane research was employed to justify increased spending on anti-marijuana law enforcement efforts. This was despite the fact that the suffocation studies were quickly contradicted by the National Center for Toxicological Research in Arkansas, which after conducting a similar but unbiased study, found no marijuana-related brain abnormalities at all.

For policymakers committed to the continuation of cannabis prohibition, the ends justify the means. By suppressing and blockading well-conducted studies, and by funding research that is tailored to provide the desired conclusions, which cast marijuana in a negative light, they gather the political resources to press for more funding to imprison and otherwise punish those who do not conform. Undoubtedly, marijuana's opponents will respond to the growing number of new scientific discoveries with more lies and more pseudoscience.

There are many examples of what happens when science is replaced by spin and propaganda. One of these occurred in February 2010, when a headline appeared on the newswire proclaiming that "Marijuana Doesn't Help Alzheimer's Disease." In this case it was sloppy journalism, along with questionable science, that was the problem. The sensational headline did not accurately represent the research it was describing. The study, as it turned out, actually had nothing to do with marijuana. The researchers merely found that HU210, a synthetic cannabinoid, had no effect on the neuropathology or behavioral disorders associated with Alzheimer's disease in mice. On the basis of those results, they concluded that we should be doubtful of the utility of that drug as a treatment for Alzheimer's disease.[51]

As mentioned before, previous studies (such as those from Scripps and Ohio State) found that THC and the synthetic cannabinoid WIN-55212-2 were uniquely effective against Alzheimer's disease. This study, however, looked at HU210—a different synthetic cannabinoid entirely—and concluded that it did not have the same effectiveness. And yet, the principal investigator of the study claimed to be advancing the state of knowledge about marijuana and Alzheimer's. "As scientists, we begin every study hoping to be able to confirm beneficial effects of potential therapies, and we hoped to confirm this for the use of medical marijuana in treating Alzheimer's disease, but we didn't see any benefit at all."[52] Without actually studying marijuana or THC, how could they? It certainly seems as if the investigators were trying to overshadow the scientific evidence on effective cannabinoids with reports on research with an ineffective one.

It is becoming more difficult to pass off biased marijuana research as solid science now that we are beginning to understand the complexity of cannabinoids and the endocannabinoid system and the diversity of diseases that respond to them. Although they develop for different reasons, there are many neurodegenerative diseases in addition to Alzheimer's that respond to the neuroprotective qualities of cannabinoids. Among these is Parkinson's disease. One study, for example, determined that "cannabinoids may prove useful in the treatment of Parkinson's disease" by inhibiting the neurotransmitter glutamate and preventing damage to neurons involved in the dopamine system.[53] This makes sense given that many patients with Parkinson's and similar diseases have positive responses to marijuana.

The cannabinoids may also have a more generally protective effect on the brain, guarding vital cells from damage and impairment. The protective quality of cannabinoids was affirmed by a study showing that "cannabidiol and delta-9-tetrahydrocannabinol are neuroprotective antioxidants." Investigators reported that the "antioxidant properties of cannabinoids suggest a therapeutic use as neuroprotective agents," and that the non-psychoactive cannabinoid "cannabidiol protected neurons to a greater degree than either the dietary antioxidants tocopherol [vitamin E] or ascorbate [vitamin C]."[54] A peer-reviewed clinical trial from the Netherlands found delta-9-THC reduced chemically-induced neuronal injury in newborn rats by 36 percent.[55] This profound reduction in brain damage led the research team to conclude that it is "conceivable that the endogenous cannabinoid system can be exploited for therapeutic interventions in these types of primarily incurable diseases."[56]

The neuroprotective effects of cannabinoids may extend to other non-pathological damage as well, such as traumatic brain injury. Studies have shown that after a traumatic injury, the brain produces a number of substances that can cause additional damage.[57] Severe head injuries automatically trigger the production of an excessive amount of neurotransmitters called glutamates. When there are too many of these chemicals in the brain, they can initiate a chain reaction of cell degradation and impairment. The cannabinoids which we find in marijuana work as effective antioxidants, potentially neutralizing the glutamate activity and stopping the cascade of neuronal damage that can follow.

There are currently no substances other than cannabinoids that effectively counteract this destructive process. Veteran cannabis researcher Raphael Mechoulam has suggested that someone who has had a stroke or head injury could benefit from an immediate dose of marijuana. The synthetic cannabinoid HU-211 may not inhibit Alzheimer's disease but it has been found to be an effective cerebroprotective agent even when administered as long as four hours following a head injury. Mechoulam and his colleagues strongly believe that "the endocannabinoids anandamide and 2-arachidonoyl glycerol, as well as some plant and synthetic cannabinoids, have neuroprotective effects following brain injury."[58] Their research indicates that certain cannabinoids, including THC, inhibit the formation of compounds (such as tumor necrosis factor) which frequently cause brain damage following head trauma. It suggests that cannabinoids protect the brain after an injury by stimulating the cannabinoid receptors into action in order to neutralize the effect of the harmful compounds. The practical implications of this new knowledge are quite provocative.

Knowing this, the National Football League might very well find it advisable to rescind its anti-marijuana policy, especially given recent investigations showing that high numbers of former college and professional football players suffer from serious levels of brain impairment due to repeated blows to the head. The intense head-to-head collisions that are characteristic of the sport often lead to a degenerative syndrome known as chronic traumatic encephalopathy (CTE). Ann McKee, a neurologist studying brain trauma at the Veteran's Hospital in Bedford, Massachusetts, has said that every professional football player she has seen has some degree of CTE.[59] Indeed, former NFL players report suffering from dementia, Alzheimer's or other memory-impairment diseases at a rate five times higher than that of the national average for their age group.[60] Ideally, NFL officials should provide players with a few inhalations from a joint, bong, pipe or vaporizer as they leave the practice and playing fields. Marijuana should be as common in the NFL locker rooms as are ice packs. If cannabinoids are the only remedy for this type of brain damage, which is an occupational hazard for professional football players, shouldn't those players be encouraged to protect themselves with marijuana? So while the NFL shamelessly persecuted him for using marijuana off the field, Heisman Trophy winner Ricky Williams is vindicated by science. According to the best data, discouraging or prohibiting football players from using marijuana is cruel and immoral and damaging to their health. The same holds true for soccer players who bounce the ball from their heads, they should be provided with marijuana or cannabis products after games and practice.

One of the most miraculous aspects of cannabinoids is that they work to protect and improve health in ways that complement one another. As we have seen, one way that cannabinoids help the body is by stimulating the cannabinoid receptors. These neuroprotective compounds, however, also work independently of that system. The usefulness of cannabinoids against both cancer and Alzheimer's disease is due as much to their synergy as to their independent effects. Researchers from the Department of Microbiology and Immunity at Virginia Commonwealth School of Medicine postulated that put together, cannabinoids and the cannabinoid receptor system may be essential parts of therapies for a huge range of neuropathologies, including conditions as diverse as Alzheimer's disease, multiple sclerosis, amyotrophic lateral sclerosis, HIV encephalitis, closed head injury, and granulomatous amebic encephalitis.[61] In the case of multiple sclerosis, there is some indication that cannabinoids not only control its symptoms but may actually slow the progression of the disease itself.[62]

The scope of the cannabinoids' therapeutic applications is almost incomprehensibly vast. The growing numbers of studies around the world are revealing just how much promise these compounds hold for an impressive array of diseases and syndromes. The British cannabinoid scientist David Pate, PhD, MSc, believes that a low-dose THC supplement could help to treat glaucoma, by reducing inflammation, increasing microcirculation and protecting cells in the eye.[63] Research is now being conducted into the possible roles of cannabinoids in the treatment of Huntington's disease, neuropathic pain, atherosclerosis, osteoporosis, diabetes and more.

Amyotrophic lateral sclerosis (ALS) is a frightening and devastating neurodegenerative illness that is diagnosed in about 5,000 people in the U.S. every year. Most commonly known as Lou Gehrig's disease (after the professional baseball player who played 2,130 consecutive games before being disabled by it), ALS degenerates and destroys the motor neurons responsible for relaying information between the brain, the spinal cord, and the muscles. As a result, ALS patients lose control of their arms, legs, and ultimately their lungs. Physicist Stephen Hawking also has ALS, but fortunately the form of the disease he suffers from progresses less rapidly than others.

ALS may be yet another neurodegenerative condition that responds to cannabis-based therapies. For example, one study of mice with ALS found that treatment with cannabinoids increased their survival rate by 56 percent.[64] In humans with ALS, this would translate to a 3-year increase in survival time. By contrast, the only FDA-approved drug for ALS (riluzole) extends survival time on average by only two months.

These hints led a team of researchers from the University of Washington to call for more clinical trials on cannabis for ALS. They stated that "it is reasonable to think that cannabis might significantly slow the progression of ALS, potentially extending life expectancy and substantially reducing the overall burden of the disease." They also explained that an effective treatment for ALS would undoubtedly require a complex drug cocktail that worked on neurotransmitters, enzymes, inflammation, and neurons—but that "remarkably, cannabis appears to have activity in all those areas."[65] After so many years of being told that marijuana is harmful to the brain, it is truly stunning and thrilling to learn that it actually protects the brain against many of the most notorious diseases.

It may also help counteract the damage done by alcohol abuse. A fascinating study found that binge-drinking adolescents who also used marijuana had less overall reduction in brain function than those binge-drinkers who did not use marijuana.[66] Brain scans of these two groups led the researchers to suggest that marijuana may protect the brain from the damage caused by alcohol poisoning. Alcohol causes brain damage and is legal. Marijuana prevents or reduces that brain damage and is illegal. It gets curiouser and curiouser. It is not as absurd as it might seem to suggest that administrators of colleges and universities take these studies seriously and require that marijuana be available at any event where alcohol is distributed. In a more rational culture, we would seize upon this information and come up with a way to use cannabis-based additives with adult beverages to guard the brain from alcohol toxicity.

A growing number of parents are discovering that giving children with Attention Deficit Hyperactivity Disorder (ADHD) moderate amounts of cannabis in capsules or baked goods greatly improves their mood and academic performance. One 16-year-old California student found marijuana to be far more effective than Ritalin. After beginning marijuana therapy under the protections provided by California's state medical marijuana law, the teen told his mother, "My brain works. I can think." His grades improved and he was elected president of his special education class.[67] Debbie and LaRayne Jeffries' book *Jeffrey's Journey* is a touching account of another parent's success in using marijuana to treat a child with serious ADHD and the DEA's attempts to thwart them. It is time that we look more closely at the ways in which cannabinoids work to harmonize the functions of the central nervous system for people with chemical imbalances.

One of the primary causes of mental and physical illnesses is the unrelenting stress that dominates much of our daily lives. The way that most of us live today, attempting to cope with overlapping stressors from jobs, money, and interpersonal relationships puts us in a state of constant alarm. This is what is known as chronic stress.

Extended periods of chronic stress damage our health by triggering the hypothalamic-pituitary-adrenal (HPA) system of the brain to stimulate production of steroid hormones. These hormones facilitate the "fight-or-flight response," and are tough on the body due to their over-stimulation of the circulatory system and their creation of chemical imbalances in the brain, gut, and other systems. Evidence abounds—both clinical and anecdotal—that chronic, unrelieved stress can cause depression, anxiety, compromised immunity, heart disease, gastrointestinal illness, and sexual dysfunction. Stress also aggravates existing maladies, such as migraines, insomnia, and skin conditions.

Some remedies that are effective at reducing the stress levels in our lives include exercise, humor, music, dance, prayer, and mediation. Could marijuana be yet another way to reduce stress and improve our health? After all, human beings have used it as a safe and effective stress-reliever for thousands of years. The symptoms of stress—depression, anxiety, migraines, indigestion, and so on—are those that also tend to respond well to the cannabinoids found in marijuana. The cannabis plant is the original balm for sore minds. Its effects can also work in harmony with other effective stress-relieving practices.

Cannabis can certainly work well in conjunction with exercise, especially outdoor activities like hiking, kayaking, or snorkeling. A puff or two can transform a nice hike into an excursion into a natural wonderland. The euphoria or "high" that comes along with marijuana use leads many people to feel profoundly inspired and uplifted. Of course, not all exercise necessarily works well with marijuana. As with all drugs, of course, its effectiveness depends on what one is doing and how much one ingests.

Marijuana and humor are also excellent companions. Marijuana frequently helps users to see things that are otherwise normal as really funny—or perhaps to understand how abnormal the things we think are normal really are. The sense of bliss and well-being that derives from activating our cannabinoid receptors with phytocannabinoids enhances our sense of humor. If laughter is the best medicine, then marijuana is a great delivery device.

Marijuana also increases our capacity to enjoy music. Listening to beautiful music is a great way to reduce stress, but listening to beautiful music while using marijuana exponentially increases the relaxation response. And numerous musicians have found that the marijuana high enhances both their creativity and performance. In his stellar biography of jazz legend Louis Armstrong, Laurence Bergreen writes:

"[Marijuana] became an integral part of [Armstrong's] life, vital to his way of thinking, but more than that, essential to his music. Louis was still on a steep curve, and his continual improving musical and vocal skills were captured on recordings made without the help of marijuana. Once Louis started using reefer regularly, he decided it helped his performing, his entire state of mind. The records he made before marijuana entered his life demonstrate that he was doing fine without it; after he began smoking, he simply got better and better."[68]

Bergreen added that marijuana's ability to give music a "three-dimensional, almost sculptural quality" helps explain its stimulating and relaxing effects on the famous musician.[69]

Since the discovery of its euphoric properties many thousands of years ago, marijuana has been used as an adjunct to prayer and meditation. Many who use it for these purposes find that marijuana acts to quiet the mind and to make it easier to appreciate what life and love have to offer. For some, such as the Sadhus, the Rastafarians, the Ethiopian Coptic Zionists, and even the Dead Heads, it is an aid for spiritual fulfillment. The euphoria induced by cannabinoids is good for the brain in and of itself, and their ability to enhance the sense of wonder and awe may be one of their greatest qualities.

If marijuana can work hand-in-hand with other stress relievers to improve psychological health, might cannabinoids also work directly against the damaging compounds generated by stress? Currently, Israeli scientists are on the cutting edge of research into the effects of cannabinoids on stress and post-traumatic stress disorder (PTSD) in soldiers. These scientists' research determined that cannabinoids may have a "wide therapeutic application" for helping people cope with difficult memories and stress-related disorders.[70] Another study reported that supplemental cannabinoids help reduce the number of stress-related hormones produced by the body.[71] Similarly, clinical trials in Germany reported that the endocannabinoid system helps to protect the gastrointestinal (GI) tract from inflammation and other disease symptoms.[72]

Though the science clearly supports the notion, it should be obvious that marijuana reduces stress. After all, doesn't the term "mellow" automatically come to mind when we think of marijuana? Mellow, according to the dictionary, means "easy-going" and "good-humored." Is it not the lack of stress that makes someone easy-going and good-humored? It makes sense that mellow and marijuana go together, since marijuana melts stress away like sun on snow.

(5)

CANNABIDIOL: THE OTHER SIDE OF THE HIGH

CANNABIS IS AN AMAZINGLY VERSATILE plant. It produces a huge number of unique compounds that work against the stress and inflammation that are at the root of many diseases. Due to its mind-altering and therapeutic qualities, tetrahydrocannabinol (THC) is the superstar of the phytocannabinoid family. Apart from THC, however, the *Cannabis sativa* plant produces more than 75 other phytocannabinoids that have not been found in any other plant. Although none of these other cannabinoids have the psychoactive properties of THC, many of them appear to have powerful effects on other parts of the body. Among the non-psychotropic phytocannabinoids, cannabidiol (CBD) has received the most attention.

Part of what makes CBD such an interesting cannabinoid is that, unlike THC and other cannabinoids, it does not produce its action by binding to an endogenous receptor (see Chapter 1). While some other cannabinoids affect cells by attaching to specific receptor sites, thereby promoting or inhibiting their activity, CBD acts indirectly on those receptors. It is more of a modulating agent. For example, CBD increases the amount of the endocannabinoid anandamide present in the body by slowing its degradation, thereby increasing its overall activity. It also works by steering THC away from the CB1 receptors, therefore reducing its psychoactivity. Like other cannabinoids, CBD does not work as well alone. For example, GW Pharmaceuticals, a British drug manufacturer, is currently manufacturing and testing a medicine derived from the cannabis plant that is composed of nearly equal parts THC and CBD.

They believe that CBD can reduce certain undesirable side-effects of THC (such as disorientation, drowsiness, and accelerated heart rate), while producing several of its own desirable effects (such as pain relief, nausea relief, and cancer protection).[73]

Raphael Mechoulam, the Israeli scientist famous for isolating the THC molecule, has been studying CBD since he first charted its chemical structure in 1962. Among the diseases that he believes it can effectively treat are diabetes, rheumatoid arthritis, epilepsy, and myocardial infarction (heart attack). Now, as researchers further investigate the structure and functions of this newly-appreciated compound, they are identifying even more of its positive effects on health. There is a growing body of evidence that CBD could help prevent the onset of diabetes in those vulnerable to the disease. Researchers working with Mechoulam, for example, found that CBD "ameliorates the manifestations of the disease" in mice with latent or early diabetes.[74] They found that while more than 86 percent of those mice who were not treated with CBD were diagnosed with diabetes, only 32 percent of those given CBD got the disease. This effect appeared to be due to CBD's ability to simultaneously reduce the amount of inflammation-causing compounds and to increase the amount of anti-inflammatory compounds in the mice.[75] Further research in this area has found that CBD protects the health of diabetic patients' hearts. An international research group found that CBD helped to reduce some negative cardiac symptoms and therefore concluded that "it may have great therapeutic potential in the treatment of diabetic complications, and perhaps other cardiovascular disorders..."[76] CBD also has the highest potency of all non-psychotropic cannabinoids against cancer of the breast, prostate, colon, and stomach in humans, as well as brain cancer and leukemia in rats.[77] According to Mechoulam and others, "the plethora of positive pharmacological effects observed with CBD makes this compound a highly attractive therapeutic entity."[78]

In addition to holding promise for preventing diabetes, CBD might also work to treat one of the worst aspects of the illness in those already afflicted. One of the few American studies of CBD led one investigator, Gregory Liou, M.D., to proclaim that CBD helps prevent diabetic retinopathy, which occurs when diabetes damages the blood vessels in the eye.[79] Diabetic retinopathy is the leading cause of blindness in adults and affects almost 16 million Americans. Despite its complete lack of psychoactivity, CBD is illegal to use and difficult to research because it comes from the same plant as THC.

The failure of researchers to follow up on a Brazilian study on CBD's strong anti-epileptic properties, for example, recently prompted Raphael Mechoulam to decry the lack of progress in developing CBD-based medicines. "[I]t seemed a very promising approach, but unfortunately, nothing has been done ever since. To the best of my knowledge, nobody has done any work with cannabidiol in the clinic with epilepsy, and I just wonder why."[80] It is a question well worth asking. By preventing the development of effective medicines, is prohibition robbing us of our birthright of health and happiness?

Despite scientists' recognition that CBD is a nontoxic and highly effective antagonist of breast cancer cells, this cannabinoid is still forbidden.[81] Against all the evidence, CBD is still classified by the federal government as a dangerous drug with no medical application. In fact, our government is so committed to the continued criminalization of cannabis that it actively works to prevent research that might show its benefits. NIDA-funded researcher Theodore Sarafian, Ph.D., admitted that research showing the effectiveness of cannabis against cancer actually makes it harder to do follow-up studies. "Funding becomes much tougher to get when we show that there isn't much harm."[82]

One of the main problems with marijuana prohibition is that it makes it difficult or impossible for researchers to legally obtain cannabis rich in CBD. It is only in the last 15 years that we have begun to understand the value of CBD—before then, few even knew it existed. CBD and THC compete for space in the chemical composition of cannabis, meaning that the more THC a plant contains, the less CBD it contains, and vice versa. Prohibition creates a large black market of marijuana cultivators, and since it is THC that produces the high that recreational users seek out, most plants are selectively bred to produce optimum levels of THC. Greater THC potency means using and transporting smaller amounts of the illegal plant, consequently the percentage of THC in illegally-grown marijuana has risen while CBD levels have declined. In fact, marijuana prohibition makes all varieties and preparations of the cannabis plant more difficult and more expensive to obtain.

Despite the charges of drug warriors that California's medical marijuana laws are merely a back door for legalization, activists and patients are teaming up with talented researchers and respected physicians to move the state to the forefront of therapeutic cannabis research and development. If, as the opposition often claims, medical marijuana is just an excuse to get high, there would be no interest in producing strains of cannabis with high concentrations of CBD. The truth, however, is just the opposite: The legitimization of medical marijuana in California has encouraged the revival of CBD-rich cannabis strains.

In Northern California, a group of scholarly activists who understand the healing potential of cannabidiol have launched Project CBD, a "not-for-profit educational service dedicated to promoting and publicizing research into the unique medical properties of Cannabidiol (CBD) and other components of the cannabis plant."[83] The goals of Project CBD include monitoring the progress of efforts to reintroduce CBD-rich cannabis strains and providing updates for patients on the supply of CBD-rich strains at specific medical marijuana dispensaries. The project also distributes a survey on CBD strains to patients, doctors, and dispensaries, which is intended to gather information about which strains have the most effective levels of CBD for treating specific disorders.

Steep Hill Lab, which occupies a nondescript one-story building on the outskirts of Oakland, California, is an independently-run testing facility for marijuana products. The lab has the tools to analyze samples for potency, chemical composition, and contamination from mold or pesticides, and has been recruited by Project CBD in order to identify cannabis strains that are rich in CBD. The lab began testing marijuana samples for CBD in early 2009, and as of mid-2010 it had identified twelve strains rich in CBD out of 9,000 samples. Eight of these strains are now being cultivated for distribution by dispensaries (unfortunately, four of the strains were lost due to the failure of growers to conserve and reproduce the source plants).

So far, the most CBD-rich strain found by the lab is "True Blueberry x OG Kush," which when grown indoors under artificial conditions contains approximately 10 percent cannabidiol and 6-7 percent THC (when grown outdoors under natural sunlight, the CBD level increases to around 14 percent). The grower is now working to produce genetically-stable seeds of this valuable strain. Another strain, called "Women's Collective Stinky Purple," was tested at 9.7 percent CBD and

1.2 percent THC. This strain has such a small amount of THC it is essentially non-psychoactive. The lab also analyzed a strain from dispensaries in Southern California known as "Pineapple Thai," which contains 5 percent CBD and 2.4 percent THC, as well as several other varieties containing around 8 percent CBD and varying low levels of THC.

Here are some of the strains identified as having significant amounts of CBD:

CBD to THC Ratio		
	CBD %	THC %
True Blueberry x OG Kush	10	7
Harlequin	8	5
Soma A-plus	5	5
Cannatonic	6	6
Cotton Candy Diesel	6	6
Women's Collective Stinky Purple	9.7	1.2
Jamaica Lion	8.9	5.6–6.5
Pineapple Thai	5	2.4
Good Medicine	9	8.2
Full Spectrum True Blueberry x OG Kush	14	6
Omrita Rx3	10	5.5
Bubble Gum Kush	5.8	4.1
Good Medicine	9	8
Sour Tsunami	10.1	6.7
Kushage	6.98	2.92
Wu#1	6.34	3.57
Phnom Penh	7.5	2.3

Dr. Jeffrey Hergenrather, President of the Society of Cannabis Clinicians, has an illuminating perspective on what patients' demand for CBD-rich marijuana means. "I am seeing many older patients who would like to try cannabis for pain, muscle spasms, insomnia, and management of various cancers. One thing that most of these cannabis-naïve patients are not interested in is 'getting high.' My hope is that

CBD-rich strains will enable them to use cannabis and get its benefit without—or with less of—the usual 'high.'"[84] The rising demand for marijuana rich in CBD should silence those who still claim that the medical marijuana movement is only about getting high.

Apart from CBD, other non-psychoactive phytocannabinoids include cannabinol (CBN), cannabichromene (CBC), cannabigerol (CBG), tetrahydrocannabivarin (THCV), tetrahydrocannabinoilic acid (THCA), cannabidiolic acid (CBDA), and cannabidivarin (CBDV). Like THC and CBD, these compounds have a broad array of protective effects on health. These include reducing inflammation, pain, and infection; protecting against seizures and spasms; encouraging bone growth; and (once again) helping prevent the spread of cancer. In addition to these compounds, the cannabis plant also generates many other unique phytochemicals which reduce inflammation, inhibit tumor formation, and help prevent the damage caused by inhaling smoke.

Although many people think it is possible to judge the quality of marijuana by smelling it, cannabinoids are in fact odorless. It is therefore entirely possible to have a strain with a powerful scent yet little potency. The enormous range of scents and flavors found in marijuana actually depends on the presence of certain kinds of phytochemicals known as terpenoids. Unlike cannabinoids, most terpenoids are not unique to the cannabis plant. That is why there are varieties of marijuana that smell like lemons, pine pitch, lavender, mint, guava, or fermented grapefruit. These other plants generate many of the same terpenoids that the cannabis plant does.

A large percentage of the essential oil found in cannabis is comprised of these terpenoids; so far 120 have been identified in the plant. Most of what we know about the terpenoid profile of cannabis comes from research intended to train drug detection dogs to locate marijuana and hashish. All varieties of the cannabis plant contain the terpenoid b-caryophyllene-epoxide, and since this chemical is rare in other plant species this is what the hounds are trained to detect. Law enforcement officials also use the widely varying terpenoid composition of seized cannabis products to help identify the product's point of origin. As researchers learn more about terpenoids in an effort to increase the effectiveness of law enforcement efforts, they also learn more about the positive health effects of the terpenoids found in cannabis. This is yet another example of research driven by the War on Drugs resulting in a serendipitous discovery about a health-guarding component of marijuana.

Thankfully, there are no restrictions on researching terpenoids since they are found in numerous plants besides cannabis. As a result, we know that the various terpenoids produced by cannabis have an impressive array of beneficial biological effects. Some of these effects are similar to the anti-carcinogenic, anti-inflammatory actions of cannabinoids and may be jointly responsible for making marijuana such a beneficial substance. Like THC and CBD, these plant compounds help protect against cancer both by slowing it down and by helping to prevent it in the first place.[85] Limonene, for example, which has a strong citrus odor, is a terpenoid commonly found in cannabis oil that has a strong anti-depressant effect due to its suppression of stress hormone production. Like THC, limonene also works against cancer in a variety of ways. A review of data published in the *Journal of Nutrition* revealed that limonene helps prevent or delay breast, skin, liver, lung, and stomach cancer in rodents.[86]

Some terpenoids also seem to have qualities that moderate the effects of using marijuana that some patients find undesirable. Linalool, citronellol, and a-terpinene have all been found to have both sedative and anti-depressant effects which may temper the anxiety that some people experience as a result of ingesting THC.[87] This could be one reason that so many medical marijuana patients prefer whole cannabis products to the legally available pure THC pill (dronabinol).

Some of these terpenoids work additionally to protect the body from the harmful by-products associated with smoking marijuana. Burning marijuana, like burning tobacco, produces toxic gases, known as polycyclic hydrocarbons that are linked to the development of lung and other cancers. Unlike tobacco, however, the cannabis plant also produces a generous amount of terpenoids which stimulate the production of enzymes that help detoxify those harmful compounds.[88]

Some terpenoids have also been shown to increase cerebral blood flow, which could be helping THC work against Alzheimer's by allowing it to reach the brain more efficiently. Other terpenoids have antimicrobial effects, which may help protect the lungs of marijuana smokers from infections.

The following table lists several of the terpenoid compounds found in cannabis and the biological activities they possess.

Terpenoid	Known Properties
B-myrcene	Analgesic, anti-inflammatory, antibiotic, antimutagenic
B-caryophyllene	anti-inflammatory, cytoprotective, antimalarial, CB2 agonist
d-limonene	immune potentiator, antidepressant, antimutagenic
linalool	sedative, antidepressant, anxiolytic, immune potentiator
pulegone	acetylcholinesterase (AChE) inhibitor, sedative, antipyretic
1,8 cineole	AchE inhibitor, stimulant, antibiotic, antiviral, anti-inflammatory, antinociceptive
a-pinene	anti-inflammatory, bronchodialator, stimulant, antibiotic, antineoplastic, AChE inhibitor
a-terpineol	sedative, antibiotic, AChE inhibitor, antioxidant, antimalarial
terpineol-4-ol	AChE inhibitor, antibiotic
p-cymene	antibiotic, AChE inhibitor

Along with cannabinoids and terpenoids, there is another group of phytochemicals produced by the cannabis plant that is beneficial for health. Unlike cannabinoids, which are found primarily in the flowers of the plant, these chemicals, flavonoids, are distributed throughout the leaves, flowers, and stems of the plant. These compounds give cannabis its pigmentation and flavor, and also seem to protect it from pests and diseases. Some researchers believe that, like terpenoids, flavonoids may enhance the beneficial effects of cannabinoids or reduce their unwanted side-effects. Twenty-three flavonoids have been identified in cannabis, and two of these—cannaflavin A and cannaflavin B—are unique to the plant.

Like cannabinoids, flavonoids have a wide range of biological activities. For many years, flavonoids' cancer-fighting ability was believed to result from their antioxidant effects. Scientists at Oregon State University, however, have found that the compounds actually "have little or no value in that role."[89] Flavonoids are metabolized so efficiently by the body that they have no chance to function as antioxidants. Instead, the body identifies them as foreign substances and quickly destroys or denatures them. This denaturing process triggers the production of a cascade of other chemicals (known as Phase II enzymes), which then also work to neutralize mutagens and carcinogens. Though they do so indirectly, flavonoids seem to share cannabinoids' ability to "induce mechanisms that help kill cancer cells and inhibit tumor invasion."[90]

Like cannabinoids, the scope of these compounds' activity is impressive. Flavonoids may also trigger biochemical reactions that protect the heart and blood vessels from damage by reducing inflammation and blood pressure. The flavonoid apigenin, for example, binds effectively to estrogen receptors and helps slow the proliferation of breast cancer caused by the sex hormone estradiol.[91] Flavonoids isolated from a Mexican strain of cannabis were also found to inhibit the formation of an enzyme linked to the development of cataracts in diabetic patients. Cannaflavin A and B, the two flavonoids found only in cannabis, have been found to have 30 times more potency against rheumatoid inflammation than aspirin. Researchers have noted that flavonoid supplement pills are unnecessary, and possibly counterproductive, since it takes relatively small amounts of flavonoids to obtain their beneficial effects. We can get all the flavonoids our bodies need from eating fruits and vegetables—and ingesting cannabis. As research on these compounds advances we will undoubtedly discover other biological activities and applications.

Because terpenoids and flavonoids are volatile (that is, they vaporize easily) they can be effectively ingested by smoking marijuana plant material. Vaporization, however, may be an even better mode of delivery. The lower temperatures required for vaporization would be less likely to degrade the active chemicals in marijuana, thereby delivering larger doses of cannabinoids, terpenoids, and flavonoids to the user.

Research on the phytochemical complex produced by the cannabis plant is still in its earliest stages. Who knows which combinations of these cannabinoids, terpenoids, and flavonoids will prove most effective for treating serious ailments? If the shackles of prohibition were removed from marijuana use and research, it would be possible to breed strains of cannabis with the most effective anti-cancer, anti-inflammatory, and neuroprotective properties. These varieties could be used for disease prevention in and of themselves, and as adjuncts to treatment for any number of illnesses from Alzheimer's disease to diabetes to various cancers. But until the laws change, we are wasting valuable time that could be spent finding ways to prevent and relieve suffering.

(6)

CANNABINOID DEPRIVATION SYNDROME

THE DISCOVERY OF THE CANNABINOID receptor system has changed our entire understanding of cannabis and its effects. In fact, from the inception of the anti-marijuana campaign of the 1930s and its subsequent prohibition until today, almost everything we believed about it was wrong. Hardly the harmful intoxicant that many once thought it was, we now know that it is a nourishing plant that can improve and prolong life.

We have already seen that cannabinoids can help bring our bodies and nervous systems into balance, but what happens when certain compounds block the interaction between endocannabinoids and their receptors, effectively depriving our bodies of sufficient cannabinoids?

It is well known that one of marijuana's most notable effects is appetite stimulation, or what is colloquially referred to as "the munchies," a compelling drive to eat and snack. Researchers studying the endocannabinoid system have found that this phenomenon is linked to the activation of the CB1 receptor in the part of the brain that regulates appetite. With the increasing incidence of obesity becoming a public health crisis, scientists have begun to explore the effect of cannabinoids on the regulation of appetite. Researchers working for the international pharmaceutical company Sanofi-Aventis, for example, began looking for chemical agents that effectively block CB1 receptor activity (known as CB1 receptor antagonists), which they reasoned could help suppress appetite and reduce compulsive eating. The company eventually developed a compound called rimonabant, which appeared to effectively inhibit the ability of cannabinoids to activate the CB1 receptor.

The European Medicines Agency (EMEA) approved rimonabant for use in Europe in mid-2006, and it was soon available in Great Britain as an over-the-counter drug available without a prescription. By early 2008, the drug was available in 56 countries. The Food and Drug Administration (FDA), however, refused to approve it for distribution in the United States due to concerns about its possible side effects. This decision was based on the recommendation of an FDA review panel, which in mid-2007 unanimously concluded that rimonabant was associated with unacceptable increases in the risk of adverse psychiatric events, suicidality, neurological problems, nausea,

Cannabis won't kill you, but a lack of cannabinoids could.

vomiting, and more. Then, in late 2008, the EMEA decided to review the drug's post-marketing data. Agreeing with the FDA's belief that the risks of rimonabant outweighed its benefits, the European regulators revoked its previous approval and suspended Sanofi-Aventis' marketing authorization for the drug.[92]

The first cannabinoid-blocking drug turned out to be a disastrous failure. An alarming number of research subjects in clinical trials around the world (which included 16,000 subjects in the U.S. alone) experienced severe neuropsychiatric side-effects including anxiety, depression, panic attacks, sleep disorders, amnesia, and psychomotor agitation leading to contusions, concussions, falls, traffic accidents, and whiplash injuries. Others had gastrointestinal symptoms and erectile dysfunction at a rate three times higher than those who had not received the drug. One patient experienced an increase in multiple sclerosis symptoms and another developed optic neuritis. Two committed suicide. Rimonabant also appeared to promote the development of neurodegenerative illnesses such as Alzheimer's disease, ALS, Parkinson's disease, and Huntington's disease.[93]

Evidence also suggested that rimonabant could increase the likelihood of colon cancer. A study at the University of Texas published in August 2008, for example, found that mice treated with a CB1 antagonist had increases in the size and number of colon polyps, which are benign tumors that can become cancerous if not removed. Conversely, the study found that treatment with endocannabinoid agonists decreased the number of polyps.[94] In other words, while blocking the cannabinoid receptor increased the likelihood of colon polyps, stimulating it decreased that likelihood. Rimonabant and marijuana may have opposite effects on the likelihood of colon cancer. This suggests that it would be wise to conduct epidemiological follow-up studies to assess the impact of rimonabant on increases in colon cancer. The damage already done by rimonabant may be beyond calculation. By 2007, before the EMEA suspended its approval, about 37,000 patients in the U.K. were using the drug. Even worse, although it is prohibited in both Europe and the U.S., rimonabant is still marketed over the Internet to unsuspecting consumers as a weight-loss drug by Indian pharmaceutical companies.

The global policing organization INTERPOL states on its Web site that "member countries remain firmly committed to their enforcement efforts against the cultivation and trafficking of cannabis products."[95] Given what we know about the beneficial nature of cannabis and the harmful effects of cannabinoid-blocking drugs, it makes little sense that the eradication efforts of INTERPOL and other law enforcement organizations are more focused on marijuana than they are on drugs that are—like rimonabant—actually proven to be dangerous.

The suppression of the endocannabinoid system has been connected to numerous health-related problems, from cognitive function and sleep cycles to digestion, sexual response, physical coordination, and overall happiness. In order to study the endocannabinoid system, scientists have selectively bred mice with a specific genetic mutation that disables the CB1 receptor. Studies of these "CB1 knockout mice" have shown that an absence of activity at the CB1 receptor has devastating effects on the physical and mental health of these animals. These effects include:

- Increased anxiety, increased susceptibility to the depressive effects of chronic stress
- Reduced responsiveness to rewarding experiences
- Reduced appetite and pronounced weight loss
- Reduced ability to forget traumatic memories
- Increased activity of the HPA axis, an area of the brain associated with stress and fear
- Increased susceptibility to neurotoxins

- Reduced ability to regenerate neurons in the hippocampus
- Reduced amounts of trophic factors (biological compounds associated with cellular growth and healing) in response to damage [96]

The CB1 knockout mice also had a greater risk of developing neurological problems (such as seizures) and had a greater overall mortality.[97] One group of researchers was somewhat mystified at the severity of the effects, going so far as to comment that "the CB1 knockout animals died suddenly without any obvious signs of disease."[98] (It is also worth noting that taranabant, another cannabinoid-blocking diet drug, manufactured by Merck, has proven to have similar negative psychiatric and GI side effects as rimonabant.)

The side-effects of cannabinoid antagonists and the results of experiments on CB1 knockout mice point to the existence of what we could call the "cannabinoid deprivation syndrome."

Cannabinoid researcher Ethan Russo, M.D., theorizes that endocannabinoid deficiency might well offer an "alternative biochemical explanation for certain disease manifestations."[99] It appears that a number of hard-to-treat diseases such as migraine headaches, fibromyalgia, and irritable bowel syndrome (IBS) may well be related to a lack of proper endocannabinoid activity—implying that supplemental cannabinoids derived from or based on marijuana could be of great value. Russo reasons that some people could be "endocannabinoid deficient," and he has labeled the syndrome Clinical Endocannabinoid Deficiency (CECD).[100] Cannabis won't kill you, but a lack of cannabinoids could.

Let's re-examine the evidence. Taking a drug that inhibits cannabinoid activity—like rimonabant—can cause agitation, anxiety, depression, vomiting, sleep disorders, suicidal tendencies, and an increase in accidents and injuries. On the other hand, drugs that increase the activity of the endocannabinoid system—like marijuana—result in euphoria, laughter, suppression of nausea, better sleep, resistance to cancer and dementia, and increased brain cell production. The implications are clear: When our cannabinoid receptors have an adequate supply of cannabinoids, we experience a heightened state of health. When they do not, we suffer from cannabinoid deprivation syndrome.

The rimonabant debacle and scientific studies have given us even more evidence that maintaining a well-nourished and active cannabinoid receptor system is vital to our health.

PART TWO

THE FALL AND RISE
OF MEDICAL MARIJUANA

$$\large\textcircled{7}$$

From Sacred Plant To Evil Weed In Just 6000 Years

T HE CANNABIS PLANT HAS BEEN utilized and revered for thousands of
years for its diverse health effects and numerous utilitarian applications. It seems that it was first cultivated in approximately 4000 B.C.E
in China close to the Hindu Kush region that was most likely the area
of its birth. Around 2300 B.C.E., the Chinese emperor-physician Shen
Nung declared cannabis to be one of the "Supreme Elixirs of Immor-
tality" and recommended it for many of the same maladies for which
people use it today. The range of products derived from this remarkable
plant—food, fuel, medicine, sacraments, textiles, and rope—seems to
have granted it a special place in human culture. Despite the fact that
cannabis has been an important part of medicine and spirituality for
so many millennia, for the last 100 years it has been irrationally prohibited. If science has not convinced us that cannabis is beneficial to
our health, then history should.

In the late 1980s, farmers tilling the earth for planting in China's
Gobi Desert uncovered an extensive 2700-year-old cemetery containing about 2500 graves. The combination of cold and dry weather and
alkaline soil conditions had worked to naturally mummify the bodies,
giving archaeologists a wealth of information about the former lives
of their owners, members of the Gushi culture. Along with the bodies
the graves also contained various artifacts such as tools, equestrian
equipment, and food including wheat, barley, and capers. In one tomb,
archaeologists discovered the skeleton of an approximately 40-year-old
male of high social status. He had been buried with a bridle, archery

equipment, a harp, and ceremonial tools typical of a shaman. At his feet was a large basket filled with over a pound and a half of high-quality marijuana.

When samples of the ancient plant material were sent to a laboratory for testing, analysts discovered that it was not a wild plant but that it had actually been cultivated. This conclusion was based on the fact that it had a higher ratio of THC to CBD than wild varieties, indicating that the cannabis had been bred for psychoactive potency. In addition, the material had been cleared of twigs and stems, which is another sign that it was used for its psychoactive properties. The archaeologists also reasoned that since the Gushi used wool for clothing and reed fiber for rope, it was unlikely that the cannabis found in the tomb was intended for other uses. Based on these results, the analysts concluded that the Gushi culture cultivated cannabis for pharmaceutical, psychoactive, and/or divinatory purposes.[101] Reverence for cannabis reached its apex in India after its introduction to the region by invading Aryan tribes. As a result of this influx,

> *The legislation in relation to marihuana was ill-advised... it branded as a menace and a crime a matter of trivial importance.*

cannabis became associated with the worship of the Hindu god Shiva, whose devotees ingest cannabis as sacramental rites. In these rituals, worshippers use the drug in several forms: *bhang* (consisting of the leaves of the plant), *ganja* (the flowering tops or buds), and *charas* (the concentrated resin). The sunny and warm climate of India enabled its inhabitants to produce potent cannabis plants which in time became integral to the medicine, spirituality, and commerce of the region. Charas (in Arabic, *hashish*) induced rapturous states of bliss and spiritual reverie in devotees while bhang and ganja were employed as medicines for many of the same illnesses that medical marijuana is used for today.

Although there is evidence that cannabis derivatives were employed as folk remedies in Europe around the 14th century, the vast bulk of European cannabis cultivation at the time was intended to produce hemp fiber, not the resinous flowers. It is now thought that the popular use of cannabis as a euphoric agent (particularly in the form of hashish) was introduced into Europe by Napoleon's troops as they returned from Egypt, where it had long been used for such purposes. By the 18th century, hashish had become particularly popular among literary figures and libertines who had developed a passion for Orientalia.

The first major western proponent of cannabis as a medicinal agent was W.B. O'Shaughnessy, a professor of chemistry at the Medical College of Calcutta, who was impressed by the many effective applications of the plant. After establishing the safety of cannabis on dogs and other animals, O'Shaughnessy began conducting trials on humans, whereupon he found it especially effective against convulsions and seizures. O'Shaughnessy's reports on his experiments eventually helped to establish cannabis products as prominent medicines in both Great Britain and the United States.

The cannabis medicines of the late 1800s and early 1900s were mostly tinctures and pills, although the raw plant material was also utilized as a remedy for toe calluses. Marijuana cigarettes were also manufactured for use by asthmatics as bronchodilators. Due to the difficulty of standardizing the potency of cannabis medicines, the impossibility of administering the drug via the newly-developed hypodermic needle, and the emergence of highly effective synthetic drugs, cannabis-based medicines eventually fell out of favor with physicians. However, they continued to be utilized for many illnesses from depression to indigestion until propaganda campaigns led to their prohibition in the early 20th century.

While middle-class, white American society was using cannabis remedies to relieve pain and psychic ills, descendants of slaves in the American South and around the Caribbean were using marijuana for their own spiritual and medicinal purposes. Migrant workers from Mexico were also bringing marijuana along with them as they traveled northward. For the Mexican laborers, marijuana was cheaper, easier to transport, and less physically devastating than alcohol. Seeing these various dark-skinned people smoking marijuana, however, frightened many European-Americans. Their fear grew even greater when media baron William Randolph Hearst launched a smear campaign touting the plant as a cause of homicidal madness. Many citizens also began associating marijuana with Chinese immigrants and the infamous opium dens.

The demonization of marijuana escalated when Harry J. Anslinger, the first Commissioner of the Federal Bureau of Narcotics (FBN) after its establishment in 1930, launched a campaign on behalf of the federal government to criminalize cannabis. At first, Anslinger was reluctant to take on such an enormous task, especially given the fact that hemp was a common weed that grew wild throughout the country—including on the grounds now occupied by the Pentagon. He soon realized, however, that federal agents left jobless after the repeal of alcohol prohibition would benefit from the continuing work generated by marijuana prohibition and the commissioner threw himself into the job with gusto.

Taking a lead from Hearst, Anslinger wrote and circulated a lurid essay entitled "Marihuana: Assassin of Youth," and tirelessly campaigned to convince the public that cannabis was an evil weed, a toxic poison that corroded the brain and led to homicidal insanity.

"How many murders, suicides, robberies, criminal assaults, holdups, burglaries, and deeds of maniacal insanity it causes each year, especially among the young, can be only conjectured," Anslinger wrote.

The first laws against marijuana were enacted at the state level in areas with large numbers of Mexican migrant workers. The laws served a dual purpose, not only demonizing and criminalizing marijuana but also making the migrant users—for whom the plant continued to be an important part of their culture—vulnerable to persecution by the police.

The federal law banning marijuana was modeled on an earlier law intended to restrict the sale of machine guns by imposing an exorbitant sales tax. Although the machine-gun tax was challenged as duplicitous in the U.S. Supreme Court, it was nevertheless upheld. With the machine-gun tax upheld, the Marihuana Tax Act of 1937 passed quickly in Congress. The American Medical Association (AMA) protested, realizing that a de facto ban on marijuana would also effectively criminalize the production, distribution, and use of cannabis-derived medicines. The protests were ignored, and when the law took effect agents from the FBN immediately began prosecuting marijuana users (referred to as "vipers" and "hemp heads") for possessing marijuana without having purchased the required tax stamp—despite the fact that the Treasury Department was not actually making the stamps available.

Since a large proportion of these arrests were being made in New York City, the city's mayor, Fiorello LaGuardia, became concerned about whether marijuana or incarceration was more harmful to his fellow citizens. LaGuardia commissioned a state-of-the-art scientific study to answer the question. The study conducted by the LaGuardia Commission took nearly four years to complete, and produced a report entitled *The Marihuana Problem in the City of New York*. The results took LaGuardia by surprise. The study refuted Anslinger's hysterical claims about associations between smoking marijuana and criminality, antisocial behavior, changes in personality, and sexual deviance. In fact, the scientific results were so striking in their invalidation of Anslinger's propaganda that one of the authors concluded that "the legislation in relation to marihuana was ill-advised... it branded as a menace and a crime a matter of trivial importance."[102]

Scientific findings meant nothing to Anslinger who denounced the conclusions of the LaGuardia Commission. He then used the significant power of his office to bully the AMA, which had previously argued against the Marihuana Tax Act, into denigrating the results of the commission and accepting his unsubstantiated propaganda as science. Anslinger's allegations that marijuana induced homicidal madness was a calculated and effective deceit. Yet he changed his strategy quickly after the passage of the Marihuana Tax Act. Concerned that his claims about links between smoking marijuana and psychosis would be used as insanity defenses by violent criminals, Anslinger began squelching the very kinds of stories that he had so vigorously promoted. Defense attorneys were already beginning to argue that their clients were not responsible for murdering people since their brains had been destroyed by marijuana.

By the 1950s, the federal campaign against marijuana had begun to cluster all illegal drugs under the umbrella term "dope." The term had long been used to refer to heroin and morphine, and despite enormous differences in their physiological effects, the mere fact that marijuana was illegal placed it in the same category. As the decade unfolded, the use of dope was increasingly depicted as a threat to the nation, a Communist plot intended to render citizens too intoxicated to resist. While just 15 years earlier government agents had portrayed marijuana as a drug that transformed men into superhuman killers, it was now seen as leaving them weak and passive, too sapped of strength and drive to survive the pending Communist onslaught. Marijuana was now much more than a demon weed; it was labeled as a threat to the very survival of the nation.

In 1948, Congress funded the establishment of the National Institute of Mental Health (NIMH) for the purpose of (among other things) directing research into illegal drugs. In the early 1960s, a young doctor named Tod Mikuriya was appointed as the director of non-classified marijuana research for the organization. When he reviewed the research grants that the agency was funding, Mikuriya was disappointed to learn that it was only "funding searches for harmful effects and detection methods and some mechanisms of action studies" but that it seemingly had "no interest in beneficial effects."[103] Interestingly, however, the research that was being done was not finding any significant physical or mental threats arising from marijuana use. Some of them, in fact, seemed to suggest that it might actually have therapeutic qualities.

As a result, and against the wishes of his superiors at NIMH, Mikuriya began advocating for the legalization of marijuana and its regulation by the FDA. Consequently he became alienated from the NIMH bureaucrats who saw no alternative apart from the status quo of prohibition. After bringing a kilogram of marijuana back to the laboratory from a field research trip, Mikuriya was pressured to leave the agency.

During his tenure at NIMH, Mikuriya photocopied every piece of research he found on marijuana. In 1973, he combined this data with material from O'Shaughnessy's earlier studies and the LaGuardia report, and published the *Marijuana Medical Papers*, an exhaustive compendium of research on the medical benefits and hazards of ingesting cannabis. His conclusion was that marijuana is not addictive and that it has numerous medical applications that deserve careful scientific study.

⑧

HIGHER LEARNING

For twenty years, from the late 1940s until the late 1960s, no meaningful research was conducted on marijuana. Apparently, the propaganda that marijuana was too dangerous a drug to be studied was effective enough to dissuade researchers from proposing clinical trials. After all, what good could come from dope?

Another reason scientists were reluctant to study cannabis was the difficulty of working with cannabinoids themselves. Isolating and distinguishing the various closely-related cannabinoids from each other was practically impossible until the development of chromatography and spectrometry. Between the lack of sufficient technology, the propaganda against the drug, and laws regulating its proper handling in the laboratory, everything seemed to conspire against legitimate cannabis research. Raphael Mechoulam explains:

> As cannabis was an illicit substance it was not readily available to most scientists. Even if obtained legally, research with it was a laboratory nightmare. In many countries special security precautions had to be undertaken. In most universities researchers could not follow the security regulations effectively and pharmaceutical companies did not want the presumed notoriety of "trying to make money out of marijuana." From a scientific point of view cannabis research had been effectively eliminated.[104]

Fortunately, this was not the case in Israel, where by 1964 Mechoulam had successfully isolated, identified, and synthesized THC and CBD. After discovering THC, the component of marijuana responsible for its euphoric effect, Mechoulam and company turned their attention toward finding out just how it made people "high."

Despite the decades of hysterical propaganda, more and more people were turning on to marijuana. Many of these were young, middle-class college students. This became a major concern for Lester Grinspoon, M.D., Professor of Psychiatry at Harvard University. From the early to mid-1960s, Grinspoon observed the increasing use of marijuana among Harvard students, and began suspecting that this "vice" was harming the nation's best and brightest minds. Convinced that this was a serious and growing problem, Grinspoon set out to conduct research on the dangers posed by marijuana, with the intent to write an authoritative paper persuading students to abstain from it in order to protect their brains.

> Regular users actually performed better on some tasks after smoking marijuana

Grinspoon reviewed all of the available literature, going back to O'Shaughnessy's work in India and Great Britain in order to build his case against marijuana. "When I began to study marihuana in 1967," he recounted, "my aim was to define scientifically the nature and degree of those dangers."[105] Of course, he was in for a surprise. "As I reviewed the scientific, medical, and lay literature, my views began to change. I came to understand that, like so many other people, I had been misinformed and mislead."[106] This experience moved Grinspoon to write the book *Marihuana Reconsidered*—instead of the anti-marijuana paper he had originally intended. Unfortunately, unlike Grinspoon, far too many people accept the propaganda against cannabis without examining the evidence.

On another part of the Harvard campus, medical student Andrew Weil was also realizing that there was a dearth of up-to-date research on marijuana's effects on humans. Weil was a precocious and ambitious student with a fascination for ethnobotany, the study of plants and their impact on human cultures. In his book *The Natural Mind*, Weil wrote: "Although thousands of articles were available on hemp (including hundreds written in English over the past century), almost none of this material had anything to say. It was a vast collection of rumor, anecdote, and second-hand accounts."[107]

The most recent research on marijuana's effects on human subjects had been conducted 20 years earlier, before the implementation of the modern scientific method which is characterized by the double-blind study. Now accepted as the hallmark of a true scientific study, this experimental approach uses placebos along with the agent being studied in order to keep the investigators ignorant as to which subjects are getting which compound. Keeping researchers in the dark minimizes the role of bias in clinical investigations.

During his final year of medical school at Harvard, Weil proposed a double-blind study of marijuana in human subjects. After wrangling with academic bureaucrats and negotiating with the Federal Bureau of Narcotics, he was finally given permission to do the research at the somewhat more courageous Boston College. Weil's study revealed that while regular marijuana users did "get high" when smoking marijuana, they were not as impaired as were those who were not accustomed to using it. He also found that regular users actually performed better on some tasks after smoking marijuana, and that the drug did have a moderate tendency to increase users' heart rates.

He also found that marijuana smoking did not affect rates of respiration, blood sugar levels, or pupil size and that the psychological effects peaked at half an hour after smoking and dissipated after three hours.[108]

At about the same time Weil was doing his research on marijuana, similar studies were being conducted at the Veteran's Administration Hospital in Palo Alto, California. According to Leo E. Hollister, M.D., the principal investigator of the study, "We found that the drug makes people happy. It makes them intoxicated and finally it makes them sleepy, which is what marijuana users have been telling us happened all the time."[109]

The year 1969 saw the elimination of the Marihuana Tax Act of 1937. Also at Harvard with Grinspoon and Weil during this epoch was the psychedelic evangelist Professor Timothy Leary. In 1965, Leary had been arrested at the Texas-Mexico border for possessing a joint and had been sentenced to 30 years for violating the Marihuana Tax Act. Leary and his attorneys argued that paying the federal tax to permit him to possess marijuana would require him to declare himself guilty of possessing marijuana—a state crime in Texas–thus constituting double jeopardy. The Supreme Court agreed. The hippie movement was in full bloom and throngs of youth were skipping toward Woodstock, and suddenly there were no federal laws against growing, selling, or using marijuana.

This was a nightmarish situation for Richard Nixon, who was just three months into his presidency when the Supreme Court essentially legalized marijuana at the federal level. The new authoritarian president would not tolerate what he considered to be inexcusable nonsense. After all, the anti-marijuana laws were among Nixon's favorite tools for repressing the youth culture's dissidents and anti-war protestors.

The Nixon administration instructed the Justice Department to concoct a new way to criminalize marijuana to replace the Marihuana Tax Act. The entire bureaucracy that had been devoted to controlling illegal drugs—within the Department of Health, Education, and Welfare—was scrapped, and authority for enforcing drug laws was given to the brand new Drug Enforcement Administration (DEA).

The administration's new law enforcement approach, the Controlled Substances Act of 1970 (CSA), "scheduled" drugs and psychoactive plant substances into several categories based on what was supposedly known about their medical uses and their potential for abuse. Because the days of legal cannabis remedies had faded into distant memories, marijuana was given the most restrictive designation—Schedule I—along with heroin and LSD. According to the new classification system, Schedule I drugs were those for which there was no legitimate medical use and which had a high risk of abuse.

Dr. Leo Hollister, who had overseen the marijuana research at the VA Hospital in Palo Alto, testified before Congress during hearings on the new scheduling act. His protest was vehement.

> I have been unable to find any scientific colleague who agrees that the scheduling of drugs in the proposed legislation makes any sense, nor have I been able to find anyone who was consulted about the proposed schedules. The unfortunate scheduling, which groups together such diverse drugs as heroin, LSD, and marihuana, perpetuates a fallacy long apparent to our youth. These drugs are not equivalent in pharmacological effects or in the danger they present to individuals and to society. On the other hand, the specious criterion of medical use places amphetamines in a much lesser category. If such scheduling of drugs is retained in the legislation which is passed, the law will become a laughing stock.[110]

Hollister was not the only one to protest the new strategy. In 1971, in order to determine the appropriateness of the Schedule I designation for marijuana, Congress commissioned a group of researchers, led by former Pennsylvania governor Raymond P. Shafer, to conduct an extensive examination of its use in the United States. Despite the fact that Nixon stacked the commission with anti-drug conservatives, including Shafer himself, the group recommended on the basis of its study that marijuana be legalized. Even Michael Sonnenreich, a prohibitionist who had helped draft the new anti-drug bill and scheduling system, concluded after reading the Shafer Commission's report that, "There's nothing the matter with this drug."[111] It was Sonnenreich who gave the report its title: "Marihuana: a Signal of Misunderstanding."

The Shafer Commission's report was a powerful repudiation of reefer madness. It opened by announcing that "previous estimates of marihuana's role in causing crime and insanity were based on erroneous information."[112] The conclusion was even more explicit, dropping a massive bomb right into the middle of Nixon's war against marijuana: "On the basis of this evaluation we believe that the criminal law is too harsh a tool to apply to personal possession even in an effort to discourage use... The actual and potential harm of

> *We found that the drug makes people happy. It makes them intoxicated and finally it makes them sleepy, which is what marijuana users have been telling us happened all the time.*

use of the drug is not great enough to justify intrusion by the criminal law into private behavior, a step which our society takes only with the greatest reluctance."[113]

Instead, the committee recommended a policy of "partial prohibition" that allowed for the private, personal use of marijuana. The proposed revisions to federal policy would also allow for the "casual distribution of small amounts of marihuana for no remuneration, or insignificant remuneration not involving profit."[114] Small fines were suggested for violations such as smoking or distributing small amounts in public.

Commissioner Shafer presented the report to Nixon on March 21,

1972, but the president remained mute on the subject until asked about it directly by a reporter. Scowling, Nixon replied:

> I met with Mr. Shafer. I have read the report, I am in disagreement. I was before I read it, and reading it did not change my mind. I oppose the legalization of marihuana and that includes its sale, its possession, and its use. I do not believe that you can have effective criminal justice based on a philosophy that something is half legal and half illegal. That is my position despite what the Commission has recommended.[115]

With that, Nixon closed the book on any further considerations involving relaxing marijuana laws. The Shafer Commission had been assembled as part of the Controlled Substances Act in order to gather evidence that would determine the appropriate schedule for marijuana. According to the evidence actually gathered, cannabis and its derivatives should have either been relocated to Schedule IV or Schedule V, the categories used for the least threatening restricted drugs, or removed from the CSA entirely. Regardless, Nixon and the Justice Department refused to reconsider their approach to marijuana. In order to maintain the status quo and the public's fear of illicit drugs, the drug warriors demanded that marijuana be kept illegal.

In the addendum to their report, the Shafer Commission noted: "Of particular significance for current research with controlled quality, quantity, and therapeutic settings, would be investigations into the treatment of glaucoma, migraine, alcoholism, and terminal cancer."[116] This was the first official acknowledgement that cannabis had medical properties since Anslinger had convinced the AMA to remove it from the U.S. Pharmacopoeia in 1942.

The findings of the Shafer Committee were so profound that a newly-established grassroots lobbying group, the National Organization for the Reform of Marijuana Laws (NORML) filed a petition with the DEA to have marijuana removed from the CSA. Despite the fact that such requests are required by law to have public hearings, the DEA rejected the petition without consideration.

(9)

Double-Blinded Trials

T HE IDENTIFICATION OF THC AS the psychoactive component of marijuana by Raphael Mechoulam opened up a whole new realm of research into its effects on human health. Unfortunately, the prevailing ideology directed most of the subsequent research toward finding harm rather than assessing and exploiting potential benefits.

Nevertheless, studies sometimes yielded surprising data. An early study done at Virginia Commonwealth University in 1975, for example, shocked scientists with its conclusion that THC "demonstrated a dose-dependent action of retarded tumor growth." [117] One might have expected the well-funded cancer division of the National Institutes of Health (NIH) to seize upon this promising data and open a line of research into how to develop effective treatments for cancer utilizing THC. Unfortunately, the healthcare bureaucrats continued to believe that supporting research on the beneficial effects of a component of marijuana would send the wrong message to young people. Therefore, the line of inquiry was terminated. The termination of research into the tumor-fighting properties of THC occurred despite the lack of safe and effective treatments for cancer. In contrast, a drug called camptothecin, derived from a Chinese tree, was considered as a chemotherapy agent until it was found to cause kidney damage. Platinum-derived drugs such as cisplatin did seem to be effective against some tumor cells, but were found to cause terrible side-effects such as intense nausea, vomiting, hair and hearing loss, and infertility. By contrast, the only side-effects of THC, aside from hunger, are euphoria, disorientation, dizziness, inconsequential acceleration of heart rate and occasional paranoia among novice users.

Despite its potential viability as an anti-tumor agent, no more federal funds were allocated for examining the benefits of THC for nearly 20 years. Instead, Congress acted to ensure that federal dollars would only go to studies intended to assess the harm of marijuana (or to find ways of detecting its use) by creating a new federal agency to direct research. The mandate for the National Institute on Drug Abuse (NIDA) was to fund research into the harms caused by controlled substances, and the agency was expressly prohibited from funding research into their potential benefits. Despite this mandate, however, NIDA studies searching for evidence of harm associated with cannabis occasionally produced—to the agency's dismay—evidence of benefit.

At about the time NIDA was created and the first chemotherapy agents were becoming available for cancer patients, word was getting around that marijuana could help prevent the severe nausea and vomiting induced by the new drugs and also could restore patients' appetites to

THC demonstrated a dose-dependent action of retarded tumor growth.

normal. Dr. Lester Grinspoon, author of *Marihuana Reconsidered*, first heard these reports when his young son Danny was undergoing a grueling course of chemotherapy for his leukemia.

The treatments were leaving Danny violently ill and vomiting into a bucket for hours. He began to refuse treatment. After hearing how marijuana relieved these side-effects, Grinspoon's wife Betsy purchased some at the local high school and helped her son smoke it before his next treatment. This time there was no nausea or vomiting and Danny shocked his mother when he asked to stop for a sandwich on their way home. Dr. Grinspoon was amazed, and immediately became an untiring advocate for medical marijuana.

Patients were once again learning what O'Shaughnessy had learned in the 1800s—that marijuana is good medicine. The most profoundly influential of these patients was Robert Randall, a young man who was going blind from untreatable glaucoma until he tried marijuana. Randall found that smoking marijuana corrected the visual disturbances caused by the unrelieved eye pressure of glaucoma. He began cultivating his own plants, and was soon arrested for producing a controlled substance. He then set a precedent for the budding medical marijuana movement when he won his freedom using a medical necessity defense in which he argued that growing marijuana was less harmful than going blind.

After his victory, Randall requested that the federal government allow him to use some of the marijuana that it grew for research purposes on NIDA's farm in Mississippi. It should have been a simple request to fulfill: the NIH already had data showing marijuana's effectiveness for relieving eye pressure, and NIDA had all the marijuana that Randall would have needed to keep from going blind. When his petition was ignored, Randall enlisted the media, who loved the David versus Goliath nature of the story. Federal health agencies immediately started passing the buck and dragging their heels, doing everything they could to avoid responding to Randall's request. When NIDA received the request, Randall was told that the agency "has got to observe its Congressional mandate in this area. We cannot extend into therapeutic evaluation."[118]

Randall was not going to let a mere Congressional mandate blind him, so he kept pushing. Eventually, a sympathetic NIDA staffer found a doctor who was willing to act as a "researcher"—with Randall as his sole subject—under a provision known as the Compassionate Investigational New Drug (IND) program. Randall's participation in the Compassionate IND program was predicated on the idea that he was being assessed for the damage the marijuana smoke was causing him.

Robert Randall was more than a patient; he was a warrior. While he could have taken his special supply of government-grown marijuana and disappeared from the spotlight, he believed it was his moral obligation to help prevent other people from going blind unnecessarily. After a series of prominent media appearances, other glaucoma patients began to seek Randall out for information on how to obtain and use marijuana.

One of these patients was Ara Crone, a grandmother who had previously never considered using marijuana. When she did try it, however, Crone found that her eye pressure had been reduced by half. Randall spoke with her doctor and convinced him to follow his lead and petition NIDA for marijuana. The doctor promptly filled out the paperwork and submitted it, but the agency stalled in processing the request until it was too late: Crone's intraocular pressure became dangerously high at which point she had to undergo surgery which failed, leaving her blind.

Randall continued to increase his public exposure as a legal marijuana user. After he dramatically savored one of his NIDA joints on television, the agency cut off his supplies. NIDA officials told Randall that by using research material on television he was violating the provisions of the Compassionate IND program. They told him he could begin using THC eye drops instead of marijuana to treat his symptoms, despite the fact that the drops had already failed. Randall once again felt that the agency was threatening to blind him, and he filed suit. He again prevailed, and NIDA promised that although it was still officially an investigational drug, Randall's marijuana supply would be treated like any other prescription drug, enabling him to use it where and when he needed it.

By the mid1970s the benefits of marijuana for severely-nauseated chemotherapy patients were becoming so widely known that a recognizable and slightly sweet odor began to linger in the air around some oncology wards. In late 1977, a young cancer patient in New Mexico named Lynn Pierson was seeking a way to get marijuana without breaking the law. He contacted Randall, who had become something of a celebrity, and together they began to petition the New Mexico legislature for help. Both citizens and legislators took up Pierson's cause with a righteous fervor and quickly passed a bill allowing the medical use of marijuana with a physician's supervision.

The federal government was not so easily swayed. When New Mexico state officials requested a supply of marijuana from NIDA, they were rudely rebuffed. Unable to access NIDA's custom-grown cannabis, they decided to use marijuana that had been confiscated by law enforcement. This strategy did not last long due to growing concerns about contamination because, as part of its efforts to reduce the supply of illegal marijuana, the American government was spraying the herbicide paraquat on Mexican cannabis fields, thereby killing the plant and possibly harming those who consumed the tainted material. Having failed to acquire safe marijuana for its patients, New Mexico altered its medical marijuana bill to read like a harm-assessment study. Lynn Pierson was the first patient enrolled in the New Mexico Controlled

Substances Therapeutic Research Act. The strategy seemed to work, and NIDA promised to provide some marijuana. Disappointingly, the agency reneged on their commitment to supply marijuana for the program, and Pierson died before receiving any.

Lynn Pierson's struggle was not futile: The New Mexico saga initiated a state-based revolution for medical marijuana. Within months of the passage of New Mexico's bill, similar legislation was enacted in Virginia, West Virginia, Montana, Texas, Iowa, and North Carolina— some of the most conservative states in the nation. As Randall wrote in his biography *Marijuana Rx,* "Every state study found marijuana safe and highly effective in reducing chemotherapy-induced vomiting. In the first half of the 1980s the states routinely reported these favorable findings to the FDA which routinely ignored the data."[119] Around this time, Randall learned that NIDA and the FDA were pushing hard to develop an effective prescription-only marijuana pill in hopes that it would put an end to requests from the state research programs for medical marijuana. Officials hoped that by developing a "marijuana pill" they would be able to avoid providing actual marijuana to any more patients.

Nabilone, the first synthetic compound based on cannabis, seemed promising until it killed off a kennel full of beagles. The federal research agencies then turned to pure synthetic THC suspended in sesame oil and delivered in a capsule. This was one of the compounds tested on Randall that had no effect on his eye pressure. Also, a capsule full of oil was not going to sit well on the stomachs of those vomiting from chemotherapy.

While the federal government was attempting to find alternatives, Randall managed to enroll yet another patient in the Compassionate IND program. NIDA officials had been stalling the application from Jim Ripple, a 65-year-old glaucoma patient, until they could produce Nabilone eye drops. When the dogs died and Nabilone research was halted, they decided that it would be better to send Ripple the marijuana than face the possibility of Randall intensifying his already-vehement media campaign against the agency.

There was great consternation at NIDA, the FDA, and the DEA about the increasing numbers of requests for marijuana from patients in state research programs. The marijuana that NIDA cultivated for research was (and still is) grown on a small five-acre plot at the University of

Mississippi, Oxford. Providing all the cancer and glaucoma patients in the state programs with marijuana would require a significant expansion of the cultivated acreage. Rather than using the brainpower and resources of the U.S. government to find a way to make that happen, officials devoted their efforts to finding a way to end requests for medical marijuana. In doing so, the needs of patients took a back seat to political expediency.

The THC capsules that researchers had developed for NIDA were proving to be vastly inferior to inhaled marijuana. The major drawback was that the onset of the drug's effects was too slow to be useful for patients suffering from acute symptoms—and when it did work, the effects were extremely variable. Whereas inhaled marijuana takes effect almost immediately, ingested marijuana needs to pass through the gut to be absorbed into the bloodstream, a process which can take over an hour and which can vary greatly from person to person. Some patients found that the drug had no effect on their symptoms, while others were disturbed by its unwanted degree of psychoactivity. When the capsules did work, the psychoactive effects were stronger than those of smoked marijuana. Yet another problem was that unlike those who smoked marijuana, patients who took the capsules were unable to titrate the dosage.

The very concept underlying the development of the THC capsule was based on ignorance. There was an unproven assumption that all of the medical benefits of marijuana (which health officials were still denying) resided solely in its psychoactive component, THC. We now know that a non-psychoactive constituent of marijuana, CBD, has its own therapeutic activity that works in synergy with THC. As noted in earlier chapters, it is likely that other compounds (such as THCV, flavonoids and terpenes) also have therapeutic activity that complements that of THC. When the THC capsules were being developed, no research had been done on how to use these compounds therapeutically. Health bureaucrats simply wanted to find a way to make the medical marijuana issue disappear. The federal government needed a solution, and fast. In July of 1979, California approved a medical marijuana bill and subsequently requested one million joints from NIDA. The THC capsule was rushed through the FDA approval process. Once the capsules were available, FDA officials began sending them to the state research programs instead of the marijuana joints that had been requested. The states that put the most legislative pressure on the agency did manage to obtain limited supplies of the government-rolled joints, but never as much as they had applied for.

In 1977, Randall and his partner Alice O'Leary joined forces with thirteen seriously ill patients and petitioned the DEA to acknowledge marijuana's medical benefits and remove it from Schedule I. The DEA ignored their request, just as it had done with NORML's earlier petition, despite the legal requirement for a public hearing. Randall and NORML decided to merge their petitions, and after several trips to the U.S. Court of Appeals, the DEA was instructed to conduct the hearings as required by law. Federal bureaucracies, however, have myriad stalling techniques available to them; the DEA managed to avoid holding the hearings for eight years. There seemed to be an institutional paranoia about giving marijuana a fair hearing.

Just Say "Know"

Despite the continued resistance of federal authorities, the mid- to late 1970s saw a gradual softening of public and political attitudes about marijuana use. The fiercely draconian state laws enacted in the 1950s were slowly undone by a wave of decriminalization reforms across the country, which moved marijuana possession from a felony charge to a misdemeanor or even an infraction. A mini-industry of marijuana paraphernalia and novelties arose as getting high became more popular and acceptable. Unfortunately, the growth in marijuana's popularity was accompanied by an increase in teenage experimentation and use.

Parents became understandably alarmed that their high school children were becoming immersed in a marijuana subculture complete with stoner comic books and cartoon-character bongs. Many of these parents banded together to oppose the liberalization of marijuana laws, believing that their kids would be less likely to get involved if the threat of incarceration was greater. These parents were operating under the mindset generated by years of baseless propaganda that declared marijuana to be a dangerous poison with no redeeming aspects. Their zeal was so great that they were blinded to the possibility that marijuana might actually have beneficial qualities.

The parents' groups found a powerful ally in the newly-elected President and First Lady. Ronald Reagan, like Nixon before him, viewed marijuana use as a symbol of unpatriotic rebellion and set out to reinvigorate Nixon's War on Drugs. First Lady Nancy Reagan adopted drug use prevention as her personal project, and began traveling the country telling audiences to "Just Say No!" At one stop, Mrs. Reagan expressed her shock and dismay when a fifth grader from Atlanta said that she had heard that smoking pot prevented cancer. Actually, we now know that marijuana just might help to prevent cancer as well as the Alzheimer's from which President Reagan suffered.

In order to justify the increased expenditures and expanding militaristic incursions into the lives of otherwise law-abiding citizens, Reagan cited the discredited and infamous monkey suffocation studies and claimed that marijuana use caused brain damage. He then poured hundreds of millions of dollars into generating marijuana pseudoscience and expanding law enforcement's power to persecute marijuana users, growers, importers and vendors.

Up to this point, the domestic marijuana market was overwhelmingly supplied with cannabis grown in Mexico and Columbia. There were some areas of the country where the growing season lasted long enough to harvest ripe, budded marijuana; Florida had its Gainesville Growers guild and there was the legendary Big Sur Holy Weed and Maui Wowie. These were cannabis strains grown from the seeds of Mexican and Columbian varieties and they needed the long, warm flowering time found in southern latitudes. In Northern California, innovative growers had hybridized these strains with plants grown from seeds imported from Afghanistan and surrounding areas that flowered earlier and were more tolerant of cool temperatures. Those cannabis plants quickly transformed three Northern California counties into the legendary Emerald Triangle and greatly increased the volume of high-grade domestically-grown marijuana on the market.

In response to these growing concerns, in 1983, Reagan launched CAMP, the Campaign Against Marijuana Cultivation which was the largest law enforcement task force in the country. CAMP turned much of the Emerald Triangle into a battleground by expanding the War on Drugs into a war on U.S. citizens with paramilitary search and destroy missions carried out from helicopters by agents with automatic weapons. For years DEA and local drug agents conspired to torment the residents of Northern California's most bucolic communities until the growers outwitted them. The CAMP efforts made it untenable for growers to cultivate outdoor crops, so, out of necessity, like other persecuted people, they went underground. Growing marijuana moved indoors, into basements, closets, spare bedrooms and eventually into warehouses.

The indoor cultivation of cannabis became something of an art crossed with a science crossed with a spiritual practice. Growing indoors eliminated the variables that limited outside-grown crops, such as cloudy days, rainfall and detection while increasing the number of harvests from one to three or more each year. By trial and error, the pioneers of indoor cannabis cultivation learned how to optimize the plant's entire environment in order to produce marijuana of maximum potency very quickly with factory-like efficiency. Much of this innovation was done in the Netherlands, where the cannabis laws are lenient but sunlight is lacking. The Dutch, along with a number of expat marijuana-loving American refugees, began to hybridize cannabis seeds to produce potent plants with a large yield that matured rapidly. Shops in Amsterdam began to sell these seeds to the public and numerous Americans became cannabis tourists who traveled to the Netherlands to enjoy a "legal" high and obtain the seeds for their own indoor gardens.

By constantly supplementing his body with cannabinoids by smoking 10 to 12 joints of legal marijuana per day Irv Rosenfeld is apparently inhibiting the growth of his tumors.

President Reagan, DEA officials and everyone involved with the drug war had apparently failed to consider the law of unintended consequences. Ironically, the Campaign Against Marijuana Production only succeeded in vastly increasing the volume and potency of cannabis cultivated in the United States. The technology allowed anyone with a small, unused space to set up a cultivation operation that could produce several ounces to a couple of pounds every three months.

Just as the Reagan Administration was expanding the War on Drugs, the National Academy of Sciences (NAS) released a report on marijuana's effect on health and society. Like Nixon's Shafer Commission report years earlier, the NAS recommended that the country's marijuana policies be changed from total to partial prohibition.

Meanwhile, Robert Randall continued to spend much of his time trying to get new patients enrolled in the Compassionate IND program. Yet as a result of the ongoing and successful efforts of government officials to stall the process, Randall was often forced to tell dying cancer patients that they would be better off buying marijuana on the street than applying to the legal IND program. It took several more years before another patient managed to enroll. Recognizing that they were in for a long fight, Randall and his partner O'Leary founded the Alliance for Cannabis Therapeutics (ACT) as a formal organization dedicated to helping patients get marijuana, and more importantly, to changing the state and federal laws that stood between their suffering and relief.

Irv Rosenfeld, a Florida stockbroker, suffers from a rare and devastating syndrome that causes sharp tumors to develop on the ends of his bones. These spur-like growths slice into and scrape away at skin and nerve tissue as they grow. In college, Rosenfeld found that smoking marijuana allowed him to sit without discomfort for longer than he could remember having ever done. Before smoking marijuana, he had to get up and shift his position often to change the pressure on the spurs. Marijuana not only eased the pain, but relaxed the tension in his muscles so that they became linber and were less likely to be damaged. In 1982, after receiving assistance from ACT, Rosenfeld began receiving his monthly canister of marijuana from NIDA, and he has worked successfully as a stockbroker handling millions of dollars in investments every day while smoking marijuana. What Rosenfeld did not expect was that the marijuana would actually impede the growth of the tumors themselves.

As cutting-edge research on marijuana tells us, by constantly supplementing his body with cannabinoids by smoking 10 to 12 joints of legal marijuana per day Rosenfeld is apparently inhibiting the growth of his tumors.

With each new patient that managed to battle their way into the Compassionate IND program, federal prohibitionists became more and more committed to eradicating the growing medical marijuana movement.

Federal agencies dedicated to maintaining cannabis prohibition and to keeping it out of the hands of the serious ill have a special skill for manipulating obscure provisions for their own benefit. The synthetic THC capsule was initially still classified as a Schedule I controlled substance and placed in the same category as marijuana. In order to get around their mandate to only study the harmful effects of controlled substances, the FDA turned to a special provision for drugs whose effects are proven but which are not yet being actively investigated. The FDA pressured the National Cancer Institute (NCI) to designate THC as a research compound under this provision, classifying it as an "investigational" compound. With this maneuver around the restrictions imposed by the Schedule I classification, NIDA began manufacturing hundreds of thousands of THC capsules, forcing them on the patients in state medical marijuana programs and blocking their access to the whole cannabis medicine that is both safer and more effective.

CASE HISTORIES

TOWARD THE END OF THE 1970s, health professionals in major urban areas were beginning to recognize the first signs of a new health crisis. In San Francisco, 29-year-old Donald Abrams, who was entering his last year of residency at the Kaiser Foundation Hospital, was seeing an increasing number of young gay male patients with lymphadenopathy (swollen lymph glands). Because Abrams was an openly-gay doctor with an interest in hematology, his colleagues at Kaiser began referring a growing number of these patients to him for treatment. Abrams would examine these men, order biopsies of the affected glands, and fail to find the cancer he expected. It was a perplexing situation.

In Los Angeles, Dr. Michael Gottlieb, a 33-year-old UCLA immunologist, had been using a newly-developed technology to assess the condition of his ailing gay male patients' immune cells. His findings concerned him. Many of the patients had few or no helper T-cells to defend against infections. When these patients began to develop *Pneumocystis carinii* pneumonia (PCP), a rare lung infection associated with immune system dysfunction, Gottlieb wrote a summary of the outbreak for a medical journal. Rather than sending it in to a peer-reviewed journal, which would have meant waiting months before it was printed, Gottlieb and his partner Dr. Joel Weisman submitted it to *Morbidity and Mortality Weekly Report (MMWR)*, an official publication of the Centers for Disease Control (CDC).

On June 5, 1981 the first reference to what was to become the AIDS pandemic appeared in MMWR:

In the period October 1980-May 1981, 5 young men, all active homosexuals, were treated for biopsy-confirmed *Pneumocystis carinii* pneumonia at 3 different hospitals in Los Angeles, California... The occurrence of *Pneumocystis* in these 5 previously healthy individuals without clinically apparent underlying immunodeficiency is unusual. The fact that these patients were all homosexuals suggests some aspect of a homosexual lifestyle or disease acquired through sexual contact and *Pneumocystis* pneumonia in this population.[120]

These were the first signs of the rapidly-growing AIDS epidemic. Around 1983, Robert Randall and Alice O'Leary's Alliance for Cannabis Therapeutics (ACT) began receiving calls from AIDS patients who were extolling the benefits of marijuana for suppressing their nausea and stimulating their appetites. He offered to help them to apply for marijuana under the Compassionate IND program, but they were dying too quickly to waste their time fighting quixotic battles for legal marijuana. Randall and O'Leary felt that the only solution was to have Congress pass legislation reclassifying marijuana into a less restrictive category that acknowledged its medical uses.

Marijuana has a currently accepted medical use in treatment in the United States.

With help from Rep. Stewart McKinney, a moderate Republican from Connecticut, ACT drafted a bill that would reschedule marijuana for medical use. The introduction of H.R. 4498 threatened to undermine the synthetic THC solution that NIDA, the FDA, and the DEA had foisted upon the state research programs. If the bill passed, these agencies would be forced to do the unthinkable: relinquish their exclusive control over marijuana to a new agency that would produce and provide thousands of patients with smokable cannabis. For years, NIDA had controlled research on marijuana to ensure that only negative data reached the public. If H.R. 4498 passed, thousands of people would stand as glaring contradictions to the prohibitionists' party line that marijuana destroyed the health and lives of its users.

In the run-up to the hearings on the bill, the FDA and the National Cancer Institute (a division of the NIH) rushed to find a way to defend against its passage. First, they began looking for a pharmaceutical company willing to quickly bring the THC capsule to market, which required them to find convincing evidence that the drug worked. In doing so, they disregarded evidence from state-supported studies comparing marijuana and THC capsules, which concluded that "the efficacy of the inhaled form is superior to the oral form," and that the "oral cannabinoid was associated with more drop-outs due to side-effects or ineffectiveness." [121]

The results of studies with synthetic THC were uniformly unimpressive. The studies found that only 10 to 20 percent of the dose in each capsule ever reached the bloodstream, and that it took two to four hours for the THC to reach peak plasma levels. The variability of THC's absorption into the bloodstream left some patients unaffected while others were reeling from disturbing psychoactive side-effects such as dizziness, anxiety, and confusion. [122] On the other hand, it was found that inhaled marijuana was rapidly absorbed into the bloodstream and could be easily titrated for dosage by taking small, intermittent puffs, thus allowing patients to attain relief without becoming incapacitated.

Despite the inferiority of concentrated synthetic THC, the FDA and the NCI pitched it to several major pharmaceutical companies. None, however, were interested in distributing such an obviously-flawed product. Finally, the FDA persuaded Unimed, a small New Jersey company that marketed over-the-counter therapeutic mouthwashes, to begin marketing the THC capsules.

Federal officials pointed to the thousands of cancer patients signed up for the state programs as evidence that a market existed for the drug, and promised to facilitate Unimed's navigation through the FDA drug approval process if it agreed to manufacture and distribute the drug. They also provided the company with the research they would need to cite on their application. Most pharmaceutical companies spend millions of dollars generating the research they need to support their New Drug Applications (NDAs). The research that the FDA, NIDA, and the NCI provided to Unimed was a lucrative, taxpayer-funded gift that saved the company millions of dollars in research expenditures. Unimed graciously accepted the FDA's corporate welfare, and in early 1982 submitted an NDA for synthetic THC under the generic name of dronabinol and the trade name Marinol.

Before dronabinol could reach the market, Unimed and the government still faced one problem: rescheduling. Synthetic THC had to be moved from Schedule I to Schedule II or lower in order to become a prescription drug. Convincing the DEA to do this was not a problem, since the agency was eager to end the medical marijuana controversy. There was, yet, another concern. The Controlled Substances Act that regulated the scheduling process did, however, allow for a challenge via public hearings. After years of being denied the legally-guaranteed review of marijuana's Schedule I designation, giving dronabinol a public hearing would give NORML and ACT an opportunity to sabotage the plan. If either or both organizations objected to the inconsistency of moving synthetic THC to Schedule II while leaving cannabis in Schedule I, it would take the government a number of years to get through the red tape.

Foreseeing nothing but trouble, DEA representatives contacted Randall and O'Leary of ACT and Kevin Zeese of NORML and offered them a deal: If they would refrain from delaying the approval of dronabinol the DEA would finally hold public hearings on rescheduling marijuana. They agreed to the deal, considering it a wise decision since neither ACT nor NORML were well-funded enough to challenge the rescheduling of dronabinol while also continuing to lobby for the Congressional rescheduling bill and suing the DEA for not holding the mandated marijuana hearings. Besides, they were not opposed to the release of dronabinol per se, as they believed it might be helpful to some (if only a few) patients. They also felt that the rescheduling bill had a good chance of winning, especially with all the data generated by the state studies of smoked cannabis. It appeared to the leaders of ACT and NORML that, after thirteen years and numerous court appearances; they would finally get a public hearing and establish a federal record of cannabis' medical properties.[123] The DEA quickly reclassified synthetic THC into Schedule II, and the FDA rushed to approve dronabinol for distribution. Unimed officials estimated that the company "contributed only about one quarter of the total research effort that secured dronabinol's entry into the U.S. market."[124] The NDA was "thin and skimpy" but was fast-tracked for approval. The FDA was eager to be able to tell Congress that there was no need for medical marijuana because patients already had the marijuana capsule. Dronabinol was approved for release to treat chemotherapy-related nausea in June 1985.

It was almost a year before the DEA finally held the marijuana rescheduling hearings it had promised to NORML and ACT. The official letter requesting the hearings written by the Deputy Administrator of the DEA to the agency's administrative law judge was dated April 1, 1986—April Fool's Day. Neither Randall nor Zeese were really optimistic about their chances in front of the DEA's own judge. But as Zeese explained, despite the obvious chance of failure, "We knew that we would be able to create a record that would keep the medical marijuana movement energized." [125]

A notice appeared in the *Federal Register* on June 24 announcing the hearings and inviting input from all interested parties. Preliminary pre-hearing sessions, which were held to determine the parameters of the scheduling challenge and to establish a format for the hearings, began in August 1986 and continued into February of the following year. NORML's original 1972 petition had requested that cannabis either be moved to Schedule V or removed from the CSA altogether. In the 1974 hearings, a federal judge had ruled that international treaty obligations prevented the movement of cannabis to Schedule V. In light of this, NORML altered the new petition to request transfer to Schedule II. Short of trying to rewrite the entire United Nations Single Convention on Narcotic Drugs, this was their only option. Yet by changing their target schedule from the less restrictive Schedule V to the far more restrictive Schedule II, NORML and ACT had been forced into a compromise. Placing marijuana in Schedule II meant agreeing that "that marijuana has a high potential for abuse and that abuse of the marijuana plant may lead to severe psychological or physical dependence." [126] Of course, none of the petitioners actually believed that marijuana resulted in "severe psychological or physical dependence," although Randall acknowledged having a physical dependence on marijuana for preserving his sight.

It was decided that the purpose of the public hearings would be to ascertain if the substance marijuana had an accepted medical use in the United States, which if true would justify its transfer from Schedule I to Schedule II. In order to answer the question, testimony would be taken by affidavit and specific witnesses would be called for cross-examination. ACT and NORML were opposed in their rescheduling efforts by the DEA, the National Federation of Parents for Drug-Free

Youth (now the National Family Partnership), and the International Association of Chiefs of Police (IACP).

The hearings were held in New Orleans, San Francisco, and Washington, D.C. from late 1987 to early 1988, and were overseen by DEA Administrative Law Judge Francis Young. Doctors, patients, researchers, and activists, sparred with prohibitionists, drug abuse counselors, drug war profiteers, and parents' groups in the arena of ideological science, with each side claiming that they alone held the truth.

Back in Congress, the medical marijuana bill H.R. 4498 had gained strong bipartisan support. Yet Democratic Representative Henry Waxman of California, Chairman of the Subcommittee on Health, refused to send the bill out of committee for a vote. Randall attributed Waxman's callous political attitude to his addiction to campaign money from pharmaceutical companies and a fear of displeasing his friends at the FDA. But this was not the only reason the bill was doomed. In March 1987, the bill's sponsor, Representative Stewart McKinney, became the first member of Congress to die of AIDS. Hopes for H.R. 4498 died with him.

While Judge Young was mulling over the massive body of data presented for and against rescheduling marijuana, Randall and the other proponents were beginning to doubt their chances for prevailing. "No one expected him to rule in our favor," Randall admitted. They assumed that the DEA's top judge would hold to the party line and find a way to deny the petition.

Then, on September 6, 1987, Randall, O'Leary, Zeese, and thousands of patients and activists were stunned and elated when Judge Young released his decision declaring that "marijuana 'has a currently accepted medical use in treatment in the United States,'" and that "it would be unreasonable, arbitrary, and capricious to find otherwise."

In his decision, Judge Young recognized that "some doctors in the United States accept marijuana as helpful" in the treatment of chemotherapy-related nausea and spasticity from multiple sclerosis or other causes. Ironically, however, he also stated that there was not enough evidence to support the use of cannabis in the treatment of glaucoma. He found that too many of the reports of marijuana's effects on the disorder came from studies of (or treatment for) Randall alone, and that they did not amount to a "preponderance of evidence" establishing "that a respectable minority of physicians accept marijuana as being useful in the treatment of glaucoma." [127] He did, however, recognize that "marijuana, in its natural form, is one of the safest therapeutically active substances known to man," and that smoked marijuana offered an "important, clear advantage over synthetic THC capsules." Young also dismissed the opposition's argument that allowing medical marijuana use "will send a wrong message" as "specious." [128]

Judge Young's decision dealt a devastating blow to the federal bulwark of medical marijuana prohibition. His opinion was a thoughtful and well-supported repudiation of the DEA's justifications for preserving marijuana's Schedule I designation. Nevertheless, an administrative law judge's decision is an advisory, not an order, and the final decision on rescheduling rested with the DEA Administrator. Randall and company hoped that such a strongly-worded decision would compel the DEA to surrender and compromise, but within weeks an official response to

> *Marijuana, in its natural form, is one of the safest therapeutically active substances known to man.*

the directive was sent from DEA headquarters to all of the state field offices declaring that "DEA counsel will be filing vigorous exception to the findings." [129]

While awaiting the DEA's justification for denying the undeniable fact that marijuana has medical benefits and few risks, Randall was contacted by a young man from Texas with AIDS who had been arrested for trying to buy marijuana. Steve L. was a Vietnam veteran who had been trying for over a year to get marijuana from the Veteran's Administration or the FDA without success. His weight had climbed from 86 to 136 pounds with the help of marijuana, and he wanted a steady supply to keep him alive as long as possible.

Randall and a sympathetic physician submitted the necessary paperwork to the FDA, and to their surprise it was quickly processed and approved. This was a rather significant change from before, when applications to the Compassionate IND program could be delayed for long periods of time. It was possible, they thought, that the FDA had been convinced by the science presented at the hearings. When the application was sent to the DEA they lost the paperwork, which was their customary procedure for processing such requests. Steve L.'s doctor resubmitted the file and again received no response from the DEA. Weeks passed, Christmas came and went, and Steve had still not received his IND marijuana. Desperate and then angry calls to the DEA went completely unanswered until a field agent in San Antonio admitted to one of Steve's caregivers that DEA administrators in Washington had instructed agents "not to be in a rush about it."[130]

On Friday, December 29, the last weekday of the year and the slowest for the news media, a day when newsrooms operate with skeleton staff and prefabricated human interest stories fill the airwaves, DEA Administrator John Lawn quietly issued his decision rejecting Judge Young's recommendation that marijuana be transferred to Schedule II designation. The reason for the DEA's obstruction of Steve L.'s marijuana supply was suddenly clear: The FDA had approved Steve L.'s application the same week that Lawn was planning to issue his decision. How could the DEA have explained approving the shipment of marijuana to an AIDS patient while officially denying that it had a medical use? Lawn knew that there would be a great deal of media attention surrounding the stories, so he refused to respond to Steve L's requests for medicine and then snuck the story of his rejection of the rescheduling decision under the newswire radar. In his 17-page rejection of the rescheduling petition, Lawn dismissed many of the studies presented as evidence as "outdated and limited."

Lawn's strategy did work: the carefully-timed rejection successfully kept the story out of the media. By the time editors and reporters were back on the job in the New Year, the news was already dominated by reports of preparation for the first war with Iraq. Lawn's decision had slipped under the radar. Once they were certain that the story would be old news, the DEA approved the shipping of marijuana to Steve L.

Refusing to reschedule marijuana for medical use was one of Lawn's last official acts with the DEA. After leaving the DEA, he took a lucrative new job as the Vice President of the New York Yankees baseball organization, and after that job, he became a representative of the alcoholic beverage industry. A career administrator without any formal training in medicine, pharmacology, or psychiatry, Lawn's decision had a profound impact on the health and welfare of thousands and perhaps millions of seriously ill citizens.

On January 25, 1990, after months of fighting and waiting, Steve L. finally received his IND cannabis. Ever the soldier, Steve had held out valiantly against his disease, determined to win one last battle. Two weeks after obtaining his medicine, Steve L. surrendered to death.

On the same day that Steve L. received his legal marijuana; police in San Francisco raided the home of Dennis Peron, a longtime marijuana dealer and gay rights activist. Peron had been caring for his partner Jonathan, who was also dying from AIDS. During the raid, Jonathan was dragged down a flight of stairs by his feet and hogtied while Peron and his foster son were held at gunpoint as narcotics agents trashed the house. Police seized a quarter pound of marijuana. It was an action that would forever change the face of medical marijuana.

⑫

KEN AND BARBIE HAVE AIDS

RANDALL AND O'LEARY STILL HAD an ever-growing number of patients with a wide variety of ailments who were contacting ACT for help getting legal marijuana. Since Judge Young's ruling, the FDA had become much more helpful and efficient in their handling of the applications, processing them in a timely manner. The DEA, however, was still losing paperwork and rejecting applications for such things as inappropriate abbreviation and inconsistent punctuation. Nonetheless, some patients and their doctors managed to be tenacious enough to wrestle the approvals out of the agency.

Two months after the death of Steve L., Randall and O'Leary began helping a young couple from Florida with AIDS who had been arrested for cultivating a small cannabis plant in their trailer. Kenny Jenks was a hemophiliac who had contracted HIV from the blood clotting factor he had received and he had unwittingly passed the virus on to his wife Barbra. They were young, poor, seriously ill, and in big trouble with the law. They were, according to Randall, "exceedingly ordinary people about to engage in an extraordinary experience." [131] Randall secured legal representation for the couple and found an AIDS specialist who was willing to fight the DEA to get them legal marijuana.

The Jenks trial became a media sensation. Sadly, they were found guilty on three felony counts, but the judge compassionately sentenced them to 500 hours of community service, to be served "by loving and caring for one another." The story was heavily covered by CNN—at the time the lone titan of cable news—and was picked up by local media across the country.

It was a public relations coup for medical marijuana activists. Kenny and Barbra were Ken and Barbie wholesome: heterosexual, monogamous, and unpretentious salt of the earth people. It was easy for people who were uncomfortable with AIDS to feel empathy for them. They traveled to New York City for appearances on morning talk shows and were featured on a segment of 60 *Minutes*.

In March of 1991, after Kenny and Barbra had endured the usual delays from the DEA and finally had their IND supplies of legal marijuana in hand, they joined Randall for a press conference to announce the launch of a new ACT project, the Marijuana/AIDS Research Service (MARS). The purpose of the organization was to provide AIDS patients and their doctors with a uniform template with which to apply to the FDA for a Compassionate IND for marijuana.

"Prior to MARS, physicians who requested IND forms from the FDA could wait for weeks or even months for the forms," Randall wrote. "When the papers did arrive there was no explanation about how to complete the 31 questions... Physicians who once struggled for hours to answer arcane FDA questions could sit with an AIDS patient, open a MARS packet, go through a checklist, and put an application in the mail in under an hour."[132] The MARS forms were promoted by Kenny and Barbra and widely distributed to AIDS organizations throughout the nation.

AIDS patients responded enthusiastically to MARS. Many gay men, who comprised the bulk of the HIV-infected population, had a profound distrust of government authority and had never believed the reefer madness propaganda. Largely citizens of the "Woodstock Nation," many of them had smoked pot, dropped acid, demonstrated against the war in Vietnam, gleefully violated anti-sodomy laws, and marched for gay liberation. There was little or no stigma associated with marijuana smoking for these patients and they were eager to use any remedy that worked. Soon dozens of MARS-generated Compassionate IND applications began arriving at the FDA and a surprising number were approved in a timely manner. Of course, once the applications reached the DEA, they were routinely lost.

Around this time, Rick Doblin, a student pursuing his Master's degree in Public Policy at Harvard's Kennedy School of Government, conducted a survey of oncologists regarding their attitudes about marijuana use among their cancer patients in order to fulfill his thesis requirements and secure evidence that a significant minority of cancer doctors accepted marijuana as a safe and effective drug.

Doblin blinded the survey with a roster of questions designed to mask the questionnaire's purpose. After tabulating the data, he was amazed by the results.

"Forty-four percent of the respondents reported having recommended the illegal use of marijuana to control emesis to at least one patient with cancer receiving chemotherapy. Almost half (48%) would prescribe marijuana in smoked form to some of their patients if it were legal." [133]

Rick Doblin was delighted with the survey's results, and his report fulfilled the requirements for his degree. Ever ambitious, Doblin consulted with his academic advisor about submitting the results to a professional medical journal for publication. He opted to submit the piece to the prestigious *Annals of Internal Medicine.* While he awaited the editor's response, Doblin began to plan the next logical step to follow the survey—a clinical trial with patients using whole marijuana instead of dronabinol. He began seeking oncologists who might be willing to conduct such research.

Although the paper was rejected, the editor asked Doblin whether he would be willing to condense the material into a letter summarizing his findings. Doblin's letter, which appeared in the *Annals* on May 1, 1991, reported that "a majority [of oncologists] thought that marijuana in smoked form should be available by prescription," a statement that generated more media furor than Doblin had imagined or hoped for. The combination of Harvard's name and the illustrious journal had infused the report with significant authority and prestige.

The power of the story was also amplified by its proximity to the publicity generated by ACT for the MARS project. Suddenly, the news was filled with reports of oncologists who wanted to prescribe smoked marijuana for their patients, and of AIDS patients who were dying without it.

After graduating from Harvard, Doblin applied for an apprenticeship at the FDA. His chances looked promising until word of his application reached the top bureaucrats at the DEA, who balked at the idea of letting a known drug policy reformer anywhere near the federal drug approval apparatus. Officials at the DEA contacted their friends at the FDA, and Doblin's application was rejected. Nonetheless, Doblin's interviews at the FDA had put him in contact with several of its newest staff members. It seemed to him that some of those officials were more dedicated to science than ideology: they were the ones who had been speeding up the Compassionate IND approvals.

In June 1991, just three months after the launch of the MARS project, Randall and the other patients receiving IND marijuana found that their monthly shipments had stopped. The reason for the interruption became clear on June 21, when Dr. James O. Mason, head of the U.S. Public Health Service (PHS) announced the closure of the Compassionate IND program. "If it's perceived that the Public Health Service is going around giving marijuana to folks, there would be a perception that this stuff can't be so bad," Mason announced. "It gives a bad signal... there's not a shred of evidence that smoking marijuana assists a person with AIDS." [134]

> *A majority [of oncologists] thought that marijuana in smoked form should be available by prescription.*

In response to Mason's abrupt announcement, Randall organized a media blitz spotlighting the IND patients in order to call attention to the callousness of the decision. AIDS activists, now well-experienced in the art of media management, immediately engaged with the issue. The phone lines of the PHS, FDA, DEA and the White House Office of National Drug Control Policy (ONDCP) were soon clogged with calls from desperate patients, confused loved ones, and angry activists. Randall later recalled that "what the agencies did not anticipate was the onslaught of public anger... This aggressive telephone battering had a profoundly corrosive effect on institutional morale." [135] The AIDS activist group ACT-UP led a "die-in" protest which closed the Health and Human Services (HHS) headquarters.

Mason's sudden unilateral decision to close the IND program had cast the ONDCP in a particularly bad light and put the agency in a difficult situation. Less than two months prior to Mason's announcement, ONDCP Assistant Director Herb Kleeber had appeared on the NBC television network's "The Today Show" to caution patients not to buy marijuana on the black market. Kleeber assured patients that "no one's been turned down in the last two years. There are over 35 such INDs on the market currently and the waiting period is less than 1 month... They can get an exception from the FDA. That's the way to go rather than go out and break the law."[136]

Mason's announcement made Kleeber and the ONDCP seem foolish at best and dishonest at worst. Many of the ONDCP staff were moved and disturbed by the desperation of the calls they were receiving and initiated a challenge to the termination of the Compassionate IND program. The resulting interagency battle forced the PHS to suspend the closure until the conflict was resolved.

Mason had planned to completely end the program, forcing Randall, the Jenkses, and the other IND recipients to switch to dronabinol despite the dearth of clinical data showing its safety or effectiveness for their diseases. The ONDCP staff felt that the PHS had betrayed the patients' trust. At the very least, they wanted NIDA to continue providing marijuana to those who had already been approved to use it, including those who had not yet received their supplies.

In a scolding letter to Mason, Ingrid Kolb, Acting Director for Demand Reduction at the ONDCP, wrote: "For HHS to treat this matter as just another bureaucratic decision is unconscionable and to me, shows an intolerable lack of compassion."[137]

With the conflict in a stalemate, the final decision was passed up to HHS Secretary Louis Sullivan. In March 1992, Sullivan decided on a compromise: The program would close, but current recipients would continue receiving NIDA marijuana for the rest of their lives or until their conditions were cured. The patients who had been approved but who had not yet received their supply—primarily people with AIDS— were prescribed dronabinol instead of marijuana. For HHS, the issue was settled. And yet, none of the bureaucrats could explain how someone with intense nausea and vomiting was supposed to swallow and keep down a capsule full of oil.

(13)

RESEARCH AND COMMERCE

WHILE THE JENKSES WERE ACCOMPANYING Robert Randall on the press tour to promote the MARS project, Dennis Peron was stewing about the raid on his home and trying to figure out how he—as a Buddhist pacifist—could get revenge against his oppressors.

Peron and his partner Jonathan had prevailed in court. Jonathan was so frail and emaciated in the courtroom that it was impossible for anyone with a heart to deny him anything that might ease his suffering. Although he was exonerated, the stress of the experience took its toll on him and two weeks after the trial, Jonathan died. "I kept thinking about how I was going to get even and I kept thinking that every AIDS patient needs pot and that is where I got the idea for a club," Peron said.[138]

He knew that if he could openly sell marijuana under the auspices of medical use, then he could humiliate the narcotics squad while simultaneously helping the ill.

Peron was not your average pot dealer. He had fallen in love with marijuana during his stint in Vietnam and after his discharge he had returned to the U.S. with a duffel bag full of Thai buds. Peron was a marijuana entrepreneur and soon established a hippie restaurant with the equivalent of a marijuana supermarket upstairs. Some of the cash from this lucrative operation was funneled into the campaigns of gay activist and politician Harvey Milk. The film *Milk* includes a short scene depicting Peron as he was in those days: lean with irregularly long hair and constantly rolling joints in the Milk campaign office. Fifteen years later, with short gray hair and a button-down collar, Peron looked more like a parish priest than a hippy radical.

His first step toward openly selling medical marijuana was to gather enough voters' signatures to qualify a "Hemp Medications" proposition for San Francisco's November, 1991 ballot. The proposition advised "the state of California and the California Medical Association to restore hemp medicinal preparations to the list of available medicines in California."

Peron's timing could not have been more fortuitous. Proposition P qualified for the ballot just days before James O. Mason's announcement that the Compassionate IND program would be closed. The conjunction of the two stories—the closure of the program and the qualification of Proposition P—created something of media frenzy.

Proposition P passed with an impressive 78% of San Francisco's voters saying yes to medical marijuana. Peron celebrated his victory by opening a small "cannabis buyer's club" loosely modeled on the Amsterdam coffee shops that sell marijuana. The business was promoted as a medical marijuana service and membership cards were issued to patients, their caregivers, and many of Peron's previous clients. Peron felt safe from prosecution. Since juries were drawn from the roster of registered voters, he reasoned, 78% of them would be sympathetic to his efforts. As word of Peron's operation spread around the community, the number of his clients grew exponentially. Ironically, the publicity surrounding the closure of the Compassionate IND program alerted thousands of AIDS patients—many of whom had never considered using marijuana—to the fact that it might help them and this just increased the number of clients coming to Peron's club.

In Florida, Barbra Jenks succumbed to AIDS on March 28, 1992, at the age of 25. Kenny continued working with ACT as long as his energy permitted until his own death on July 19, 1993, at the age of 31. And then there were two less people to burden NIDA for their precious supplies of marijuana.

San Francisco was overwhelmingly affected by the AIDS crisis. It is a city that has uniquely welcomed gays and lesbians as integral parts of its family, community, and business life, and as a result disproportionate numbers of its citizens were dying.

Donald Abrams was right in the middle of this growing epidemic.

Since seeing some of the first signs of the disease—cases of swollen lymph glands in gay men—Donald Abrams had steered his career away from clinical oncology and toward working with AIDS. He helped to establish Ward 86, the world's first dedicated AIDS ward, at San Francisco General Hospital where he became the Assistant Director of the AIDS Program. He soon realized that he was helping to make medical history. When Harold Varmus of the NIH requested that medical professionals find a name for the agent causing AIDS (since "acquired immunodeficiency syndrome" did not describe the underlying cause), it was Abrams who suggested "human immunodeficiency virus," or HIV.

As the epidemic spread, increasing numbers of HIV patients were reporting that smoking or eating marijuana was helping them with their symptoms. Abrams' own partner who had suffered from the illness, smoked marijuana every day and had outlived the members of three support groups without using conventional medications.

I kept thinking about how I was going to get even and I kept thinking that every AIDS patient needs pot and that is where I got the idea for a club.

At SFGH's Ward 86, "Brownie" Mary Rathbun was the volunteer of the year for two years running. Brownie Mary was a tough and irreverent 70-year-old who ran errands for nurses and patients and brought her "kids"—the young men with AIDS—marijuana-laced brownies to ease their suffering and jump-start their appetites. The staff both knew and approved of her activities; the brownies increased patients' appetites and seemed to ease their anxiety over their impending deaths. The staff also appreciated the nonmedicinal pastries she brought for them.

In the summer of 1992, while Brownie Mary was baking a batch of brownies at a friend's home in Sonoma County just north of San Francisco, she was interrupted by the sheriff who stopped by looking for another marijuana suspect. When he saw the quarter pound of sifted marijuana Mary was about to fold into the batter, he arrested her. Since Mary had brought the marijuana with her from San Francisco, she was charged with felonious transportation of a controlled substance.

Dennis Peron and Brownie Mary had been buddies for years, and he had often helped her obtain the marijuana she used for her medicinal baking. He was the first person Mary called after her arrest, and he immediately realized the enormity of the story. The arrest of a little old lady for baking marijuana brownies for patients with AIDS was the ultimate human interest story. Peron alerted every media outlet he knew, and they eagerly embraced the story. CNN pounced on the story and produced an extremely sympathetic segment which was broadcast internationally and put in heavy rotation. Brownie Mary was defiant and unapologetic; vowing to keep giving her kids brownies until she was jailed.

In July 1992, HIV experts from around the world gathered in Amsterdam for the International AIDS Conference. There had not been any significant advances in HIV treatments, making many of the lectures and panel discussions seem pointlessly vacuous, so Donald Abrams decided to peruse the poster displays instead. One poster caught his attention. It summarized the findings of a study conducted by a team at UCSF, which included his colleague Marcus Conant, M.D., entitled "Dronabinol [Marinol] Stimulates Appetite and Weight Gain in HIV Patients." Abrams was troubled by the study, which had found that a full quarter of patients had withdrawn "due to suspected adverse effects of study medication." [139] He felt that it was oddly appropriate that a study on dronabinol (synthetic THC) was being presented in Amsterdam, a nation famous for its relaxed attitudes about cannabis use.

> *If the narcs think I'm going to stop baking pot brownies for my kids with AIDS, they can go fuck themselves in Macy's window!*

While in his hotel room, Abrams turned on the television, flipped to the news, and was astounded to see Brownie Mary on CNN. It was bizarre: He was on the other side of the world, and he was watching Ward 86's volunteer of the year on television. When he learned that she had been arrested for baking brownies, the experience became even more surreal.

Back in the U.S., Rick Doblin was also watching the Brownie Mary saga unfold on TV. After graduating from Harvard, Doblin had founded the Multidisciplinary Association for Psychedelic Studies (MAPS) to

encourage and facilitate clinical research into the therapeutic applications of controlled substances. Since conducting his survey of oncologists' attitudes about marijuana use, Doblin had been trying to find a
doctor willing to conduct a clinical trial with patients using cannabis.
He felt that, since the DEA had refused to follow their own judge's recommendation to reschedule marijuana, the only way to change how
marijuana was dealt with was to establish a body of scientific evidence
that would be acceptable to the FDA.

Doblin drafted a "to whom it may concern" letter and sent it to
the AIDS program at SFGH. He suggested that since the hospital was
"Brownie Mary's institution," it was appropriate that a study of marijuana's effect on AIDS wasting syndrome be conducted there. The letter
was directed to Abrams because he was investigating unapproved and
alternative AIDS medications in use by the HIV community. Abrams
had seen the benefits of marijuana, but he had not seen any evidence
of serious harm (as he had with alcohol, cigarettes, and any number
of prescription drugs he had at his disposal). With so many patients
using medical marijuana, he felt it was important to gather more data
about it in case there was, in fact, some unidentified risk. NIDA, for
example, had been making assertions for nearly 20 years—based on
evidence drawn from well-funded pseudoscientific studies—that marijuana damaged the immune system.

Abrams contacted Doblin, and they began collaborating on a protocol for a study of marijuana in the treatment of AIDS wasting syndrome.
Doblin first suggested using marijuana brownies but that approach was
discarded over concerns about standardizing potency and preventing spoilage. The revised study proposed to compare patients taking
dronabinol, patients smoking marijuana, and patients using neither to
determine whether they experienced positive weight gain. Abrams and
Doblin consulted with researchers at the FDA and ushered the protocol
through approval from hospital committees, state and university institutional review boards, and the FDA. However, the study hit a road-
block at NIDA—which was still the only legal source for marijuana for
research in the country—when the agency refused to provide Abrams
with the marijuana he needed to conduct the trial.

While Abrams and Doblin were battling NIDA, the San Francisco Board of Supervisors voted to pass a measure making medical

marijuana the lowest priority for law enforcement and also declared a "Brownie Mary Day" in San Francisco. A rally was held for her and from a stage set up in front of city hall, Brownie Mary defiantly vowed, "If the narcs think I'm going to stop baking pot brownies for my kids with AIDS, they can go fuck themselves in Macy's window!" Brownie Mary had become something of a folk hero, and the charges against her were dropped.

As support for medical marijuana grew, so did its use. Dennis Peron moved his buyer's club from the studio apartment it had occupied to a large former dance studio located near one of the city's primary public transportation hubs, and soon afterward he invited the media to take a first-hand look at his operation. Buyer's clubs soon began appearing in other locations including New York, Seattle, and Key West.

Initiatives modeled on Proposition P were quickly passed in cities and communities across California. This wave of public support for medical marijuana motivated California state legislators to pass a measure reclassifying marijuana as a Schedule II drug in the state, enabling it to be made available by prescription. Governor Pete Wilson vetoed the bill, however, correctly noting that state law could not make a drug available by prescription nor could it reschedule a controlled substance.

Dealing with NIDA was a uniquely unpleasant experience for Abrams. For nine full months, Abrams had asked NIDA officials about the status of his request and was repeatedly rebuffed with assurances and apologies. In April 1995, NIDA Director Alan Leshner, Ph.D., informed Abrams that "we cannot comply with your request" because "the study was flawed" and he "couldn't justify using our scarce resources." [140]

Abrams was infuriated, and responded with a scathing letter:

> To receive the first communication from your office nine months after we sent the initial submission is offensive and insulting... The apparent absence of any possibility to discuss your concerns and to modify the protocol so that we may be able to work together for the benefit of our patients is also unacceptable in my opinion... Your concerns about the scientific merit of the study have not been shared by a number of competent reviewers and investigators...
>
> Finally the sincerity with which you share my "hope that new treatments will be found swiftly" feels so hypocritical that it makes

me cringe… You and your Institution had an opportunity to do a service to the community of people living with AIDS. You and your Institution failed. In the words of the AIDS activist community: SHAME![141]

It was a critical moment for the medical marijuana movement. A confluence of political deception, scientific frustration, and grassroots activism were generating powerful momentum for reform. Activists used Leshner's rejection and Abram's response as weapons in an increasingly intense public relations battle.

You and your Institution had an opportunity to do a service to the community of people living with AIDS. You and your Institution failed. In the words of the AIDS activist community: SHAME!

Shortly after NIDA's refusal to permit Doblin and Abrams' study, the California legislature passed a bill exempting medical marijuana users from prosecution under state law. Just as he had with the state rescheduling measure, Governor Wilson vetoed the bill. This time, he decided to pass the buck: "The Clinton Administration said in August marijuana should not be used for any purpose," he said, referring to Attorney General Janet Reno's cruel refusal to call a moratorium on the arrest of medical marijuana patients.

Although Dennis Peron had initially modeled his buyer's club on Dutch "coffee shops," his operation soon dwarfed anything found in the Netherlands. He moved out of the old dance studio and relocated to a massive five-story building on Market Street in San Francisco that was just a short walk from City Hall. The Cannabis Buyers' Club (CBC) was truly a phenomenon. Never before had anyone anywhere sold so much marijuana so openly. Along with the Golden Gate Bridge and Fisherman's Wharf, the club became a regular sight-seeing attraction for tour buses It was a wonderful operation that created a de facto community center for a lot of down-and-out people with serious illnesses who had previously been isolated shut-ins. The CBC provided meeting spaces and lounges with comfortable seating and big-screen

TVs. Affordable (and free) on-site housing was provided for workers who were also patients. The club even had its own softball team. There were support groups for cannabis users with various illnesses, as well as for those in recovery from dangerous drugs like alcohol and heroin. It was beautiful.

The first floor of the CBC building contained an intake center, where patients would be screened, as well as a number of meeting rooms. A large freight elevator transported club members with movement restrictions up to the other floors.

The second floor contained Peron's office, which overlooked the front of the club and Market Street. It was there that he met with patients, activists, reporters and sycophants from around the globe and conspired to launch Proposition 215, the grass-roots campaign that ignited the medical marijuana revolution. The floor also included a pleasant dorm-style living area with a sleek kitchen and living room. Behind some of the panels on this floor, as in some haunted mansion, were concealed rooms where much of the best cannabis was secured.

The third floor housed the "Mexican Bar," where lower-grade marijuana was sold, as well as the "Brownie Mary Edibles Bar." The fourth floor housed the "California Bar," where the top-grade marijuana was sold, and lounging areas and a performance space that that hosted a number of fundraisers for the Proposition 215 campaign and various legal battles. The fifth and uppermost floor was where the marijuana was examined, bought, and packaged, and was restricted to a few authorized employees. From the long table where thousands of baggies were filled with medical marijuana, one could see the impressive dome of City Hall. Many dedicated citizens worked under that dome—including Terence Hallinan, Angela Alioto, Sue Bierman, Tom Ammiano, and others—who understood that marijuana was a powerful medicine that profoundly helped people with AIDS, cancer and other misery-inducing illnesses. These public servants were, like Abrams, Peron, Randall, and other activists, standing up to federal tyranny in defense of the voiceless thousands who simply wanted to feel better. Standing in Peron's club, staring at the dome of City Hall, it was easy to feel that all around you history was being made. By the time the Market Street CBC opened its doors, it was serving over 10,000 members.

It was well known that one did not have to be deathly ill to get a CBC membership and Peron's club was raided and ultimately closed due to the loose admission standards. For the most part, however, politicians in San Francisco defended the club because they felt that if non-patients were getting marijuana from the club safely, instead of from the street, then perhaps that was not such a bad trade off for making the medicine easily available to the seriously ill. In addition to being a revolutionary distribution center for patients in need of medicine, the CBC was also the launching pad for a series of political reforms that would change the face of marijuana policy in California and beyond. It was from there that a network of activists, patients, and medical marijuana suppliers conceived of a ballot initiative to enact a state law that would protect patients from arrest. In order to do so, they took advantage of California's unique ballot initiative process, which allows citizens to enact or repeal laws that legislators have failed to address satisfactorily. In the Fall of 1995, activists began gathering signatures to qualify a medical marijuana proposition for the 1996 election. The effort succeeded—following an infusion of cash from a group of wealthy sympathizers—and the campaign for Proposition 215 began.

GRASS ROOTS VICTORY

A LAN LESHNER WAS IN A difficult situation as the director of NIDA.
The agency's mandate was to "develop and conduct comprehensive health education, training, research, and planning programs for the prevention and treatment of drug abuse and for the rehabilitation of drug abusers."[142] With its emphasis on drug *abuse* rather than drug *use*, NIDA was by definition prohibited from facilitating research into the benefits of restricted substances. Leshner was in no position to contradict this directive. If he had, he and his organization—and by extension the entire Clinton administration—would likely have been the targets of an intense political assault.

Rather than continuing to play the role of the bureaucratic villain and take the heat of public disapproval, Leshner decided to make NIDA's parent agency, the NIH, responsible for deciding if studies with therapeutic marijuana should be approved. He agreed to provide marijuana for any study that passed the NIH peer review process.

Donald Abrams hoped that Leshner's decision would help to neutralize the political bias that had been frustrating his attempts to begin the marijuana/dronabinol study.

He submitted a new protocol incorporating the corrections that NIDA reviewers had suggested after their previous rejection of the study, such as having the research subjects remain at the study site at SFGH rather than taking their marijuana home.

Abrams was somewhat surprised when, in August, just three months before Californians would vote on Proposition 215, he received yet another rejection notice, this time from the NIH. When the peer review panel's comments arrived, he began to understand the extent to which a reefer madness bias still influenced official attitudes towards marijuana. Abrams wrote:

> Two of the three reviewers mentioned in their comments that they were unclear as to why the Consortium investigators would choose to conduct a trial with such a "toxic" substance. The final reviewer was concerned that if patients with AIDS wasting developed increased appetite following marijuana ingestion... that they may subsequently develop hyperlipidemia (high cholesterol and triglycerides) and atherosclerosis. The peer review panel seemed to have missed the point: the reason the substance was being studied was because it was being so widely used in the local community. The reviewers' apparent lack of insight into the natural history of the HIV-wasting syndrome also was of concern to the once again defeated protocol team.[143]

The government is saying there are no scientific studies proving the medical benefits of marijuana, but they're also not letting the studies be conducted.

The rejection of the second proposal came at a time when the federal government was intensifying its resistance to the medical marijuana movement. As part of this renewed assault, the government sent its drug czar, General Barry McCaffrey, to California and Arizona (which was getting ready to vote on a measure even more radical than California's Proposition 215) to campaign against the medical marijuana initiatives on the ballot in those states. During his tour, McCaffrey repeatedly asserted that "there is not a shred of scientific evidence that shows that smoked marijuana is useful or needed. This is a cruel hoax that sounds more like something out of a Cheech and Chong show."[144] These were the federal talking points: "not a shred of evidence," "cruel hoax," and "Cheech and Chong show." The retired general's argument lacked scientific authority, especially when juxtaposed with a world-class AIDS researcher's exasperated complaint that, "The government is saying there are no scientific studies proving the medical benefits of marijuana, but they're also not letting the studies be conducted."[145] Activism and science had collided and merged into a political force. Activists insisted that marijuana was a good medicine that helped keep people alive. The government insisted that it was dangerous and that there was no evidence it helped anyone. Scientists responded that they were not being allowed to do the research to find the evidence. The government's duplicity had become embarrassingly obvious.

California's Proposition 215 passed on Election Day in 1996 with 56 percent of the vote. It was a decisive victory and a powerful indictment of the government's unwillingness to deal honestly with the issue. Arizona's more sweeping measure, which allowed for the medical use of all Schedule I drugs, easily passed with 65 percent of the vote. It was a humiliating loss for prohibitionists and the drug war industry. Even Arizona—traditionally a conservative state—had given them the finger.

Rather than heeding the will of the voters and redirecting their actions toward treating medical marijuana scientifically and compassionately, federal authorities instead decided to try to crush the movement. In response to what they perceived to be a veritable uprising, the government initiated an ill-considered, ham-handed pogrom aimed at doctors and patients alike. McCaffrey and other opponents of reform insulted California and Arizona voters by saying that they had been "asleep at the switch" on Election Day, or that they had been duped by pro-drug millionaires. At a funereally grim press conference, Attorney General Janet Reno, flanked by McCaffrey, NIDA director Leshner, and HHS Secretary Donna Shalala, threatened that "U.S. attorneys in both states will continue to review cases for prosecution and DEA officials will review cases, as they have, to determine whether to revoke the registration of any physician who recommends or prescribes so-called Schedule I substances" and that doctors might face "further enforcement action."[146]

The sullen and punitive nature of the press conference clearly illustrated the government's brutal indifference to the plight of the seriously ill in the face of a threat to federal drug policy. The outcry against the announcement was swift, massive, and seething. The public, physicians, and their professional organizations were outraged. Editorials across the nation decried the Attorney General's threats as an interference with the doctor-patient relationship. A group of San Francisco doctors and patients responded by filing a class-action suit against Reno,

McCaffrey, and DEA Administrator Thomas Constantine for violating the First Amendment.

The public reaction was so intense that within a week McCaffrey had retreated from his "not a shred of evidence" comments and announced a $1 million review of scientific evidence on medical marijuana to be conducted by the National Academy of Sciences' Institute of Medicine (IOM). The government had used this tactic to appease reformers in the past—a similar review had been done by the same body in 1981. The earlier report had confirmed marijuana's usefulness in treating a variety of physical and psychological illnesses. The government could have saved $1 million by simply reviewing those findings. Uncovering the truth was not, however, the government's real priority; the actual goal was to preserve the enormous drug war bureaucracy.

The NIH also rushed to conduct a two-day workshop on medical marijuana, the content of which likewise undermined the drug czar's simple-minded Cheech and Chong rhetoric. Rick Doblin, who attended the workshop and was still promoting Abrams' efforts to conduct research, assured him that "NIDA, the NIH, and the Clinton Administration will have a very difficult time convincing the press that the publicly-announced new openness to research is more than a PR front and delay tactic if your next NIH grant gets rejected."[147]

In California, the state politicians watched the government's war on medical marijuana research unfold, and they resented it. The legislature was not about to wait around for NIDA and the DEA to remove the research blockade, so in 2000 it established an agency to fund clinical trials of marijuana's alleged benefits. The new agency, the Center for Medical Cannabis Research (CMCR), was administered through the University of California and granted $8.7 million in funds. Though the actual marijuana for the studies would still have to come from NIDA, it was thought that the authority of the State of California would help expedite the process. As it turned out, the state was indeed able to put a lot more pressure on the government than individual research teams could.

During 1996 new types of HIV treatments were released and for the first time since the initial AIDS cases appeared, there was hope for the patients. The drugs, protease inhibitors, interfered with the HIV's ability to replicate and worked quickly to bring some of the sickest patients back from the threshold of death. Unfortunately, the side-effects were often brutal: chronic nausea, diarrhea, and headaches. Using marijuana to combat these problems often allowed people with AIDS to adhere to their medication régime more comfortably and effectively.

In January 1997, Abrams scheduled a meeting with Leshner at NIDA's headquarters to discuss the barriers to researching marijuana's benefits. Leshner emphasized to Abrams that NIDA was "the National Institute *on* Drug Abuse, not *for* Drug Abuse" and could not supply marijuana to studies seeking a beneficial result.[148] Consequently, Abrams and his team devised a new study protocol, this time exploring the potential *harm* that marijuana or dronabinol might cause by interacting with the new protease inhibitor AIDS drugs. Although the study was designed and pitched as a harm-assessment study, it would also measure weight gain and other factors that might indicate therapeutic benefits. The clinical trial was a Trojan horse, finally allowing researchers to get the data they had been seeking for years.

Now Abrams was playing the game. Reviewers gave the submission special attention, and the study was promptly approved. The first patients were enrolled on May 12, 1998, when they began a 25-day stay in the research wing of SFGH during which they were randomly selected to receive dronabinol, a placebo, or 3.95% THC cannabis cigarettes—courtesy of NIDA.

⑮

GOVERNMENT WASTE

CALIFORNIA'S ATTORNEY GENERAL DAN LUNDGREN vowed to interpret Proposition 215 in the most restrictive manner possible. He harassed Peron in the courts until he managed to get a ruling to close the Cannabis Buyers Club, which was by then serving thousands of patients each day. Peron managed to avoid prison time, and moved to a farm in the northern part of the state to cultivate organic cannabis with a collective of fellow patients. When Lundgren decided to run for governor after his term as Attorney General had expired, Peron jumped into the Republican primary as his opponent. Neither of them was elected governor, but Lundgren's replacement as Attorney General, Bill Lockyer, was less hostile to medical marijuana than his predecessor, and dispensaries, based on Peron's model began proliferating throughout the state.

One of these was opened by Jeff Jones, a Midwesterner who had relocated to the Bay Area to join the medical marijuana revolution. Located in an economically-depressed part of downtown Oakland, across the bay from San Francisco, the dispensary looked more like a pharmacy than a community center. Patients' paperwork confirming their physician's recommendation was meticulously verified, and smoking was not permitted on site. Jones' dispensary did not provide the kind of arena for socializing that the CBC had, but its seriousness and sobriety did provide a needed counterbalance to Peron's freewheeling leniency. As part of their investigation, members of the IOM medical marijuana review group visited Jones' club, as well as the CBC and two other clubs where they got a first-hand view of how these dispensaries were trying to turn a black market operation into a legitimate medical enterprise.

The IOM group's $1 million final report was a complete repudiation of General McCaffrey's assertion that there was no evidence pointing to marijuana's medical value:

> The accumulated data suggest a variety of indications, particularly for pain relief, antiemesis, and appetite stimulation. For patients such as those with AIDS or who are undergoing chemotherapy, and who suffer simultaneously from severe pain, nausea, and appetite loss, cannabinoid drugs might offer a broad spectrum of relief not found in any other single medication. The data are weaker for muscle spasticity but moderately promising. The least promising categories are movement disorders, epilepsy, and glaucoma... The therapeutic effects of cannabinoids are most well established for THC... But it does not follow from this that smoking marijuana is good medicine.[149]

Despite the group's understandable reservations about delivering therapeutic compounds via smoking, they acknowledged that marijuana offered unique relief to desperately ill patients. They recommended "short-term use of smoked marijuana (less than six months) for patients with debilitating symptoms (such as intractable pain or vomiting)." They also commented about the need to develop alternative delivery systems.

"Until a nonsmoked rapid-onset cannabinoid drug delivery system becomes available, we acknowledge that there is no clear alternative for people suffering from *chronic* conditions that might be relieved by smoking marijuana such as pain or AIDS wasting."[150] Without knowing the history of the government's attitudes toward medical marijuana, one might have expected the officials at NIDA, the DEA, and the NIH to take the IOM's advice seriously (they had, after all, devoted $1 million to the study) and begin providing seriously ill patients with marijuana. Among other things, they could have immediately reopened the Compassionate IND program.

Instead, the federal government became even more committed to eradicating the fledgling medical marijuana industry, and began bludgeoning it with lawsuits.

Having learned that the public overwhelmingly supported medical marijuana and that raiding the dispensaries had been a terrible PR move, the Justice Department filed a series lawsuits intended to shut down clubs in Oakland, San Francisco, and Los Angeles. Peron's club had already been closed by the state courts and the rest capitulated—except for Jeff Jones' Oakland dispensary. He was strictly professional. He knew he was following the IOM's recommendations, and was confident enough to battle the government in court.

Jones' case went all the way to the Supreme Court, and although he lost in 2001, the resulting attention generated even more public sympathy for the cause. Every time the government won a court case, they lost in the arena of public opinion. The federal officials' intransigence in the face of their own expert panel's directive aggravated the public. Cancer, AIDS, and chronic pain were challenges that everyone had dealt with, either themselves or their friends or family, and it was widely recognized that compared to many prescription drugs, marijuana was relatively harmless.

For patients such as those with AIDS or who are undergoing chemotherapy, and who suffer simultaneously from severe pain, nausea, and appetite loss, cannabinoid drugs might offer a broad spectrum of relief not found in any other single medication.

As is so often the case, California led the way and soon other states were moving toward legalizing medical marijuana. Some activist groups were preparing ballot initiatives, while others were lobbying their state representatives to take a stand for patients. In 1998, Washington, Oregon, and Alaska enacted legislation to protect medical marijuana users. In 2000, Hawaii, Colorado, and Nevada joined the movement toward justice and compassion.

The reputations of McCaffrey and the DEA were trashed by their responses to the state initiatives. The DEA appeared to be rigid, fossilized and arrogant with a sense of bureaucratic self-importance. Almost no one continued to believe their hype about medical marijuana. The agency was becoming increasingly discredited for being deceitful and out of touch as state after state said yes to medical marijuana.

The IOM report helped to spur the development of safer and more effective ways of delivering the protective compounds in marijuana. Its conclusions praised the uniquely therapeutic value of the cannabinoids while dismissing smoking as an effective method for ingesting them. It acknowledged the need for patients to get the positive aspects of smoking—effective titration and rapid onset—without having to inhale the undesirable byproducts of combustion. The report's suggestion that "a nonsmoked rapid-onset cannabinoid drug delivery system" needed to be developed was taken seriously by enterprising innovators, who began to reinvent the way people use marijuana.

Prior to the release of the IOM report, some cannabis users had already been experimenting with ways to vaporize the active ingredients without combusting the plant material. The first models of vaporizers were imprecise and often singed the material instead of vaporizing it. For a while, heat guns (used for removing paint from surfaces) were used, but they were too heavy and awkward for use as anything other than a novelty device.

Until a nonsmoked rapid-onset cannabinoid drug delivery system becomes available, we acknowledge that there is no clear alternative for people suffering from chronic *conditions that might be relieved by smoking marijuana such as pain or AIDS wasting.*

Soon a German company, Storz & Bickel, engineered a novel way to effectively deliver a pure mist of cannabinoids and terpenes without the noxious combustion gases. The "Volcano" was designed to blow heated air through ground marijuana, pushing the resulting vapor into a plastic balloon from which the user then inhales the smoke-free cannabinoids. Despite its comparatively high price—about 10 times the cost of a good glass bong—the Volcano quickly became the vaporizer of choice. As a result, when Donald Abrams proposed a study comparing smoked and vaporized marijuana, he decided to use the Volcano.

In Great Britain, where marijuana had become a popular remedy for a large number of MS patients, the small drug company GW

Pharmaceuticals set out to develop a natural cannabinoid complex drug that could be ingested effectively without smoking. In order to do so, the company's founder, Geoffrey Guy, M.D., managed to secure permission from the British government to begin cultivating cannabis. GW Pharmaceuticals cultivated the plant from standardized strains, extracted the plant's naturally-occurring cannabinoids, and concentrated them for use in an oral spray. By allowing the active components of cannabis to be absorbed sublingually, this method of delivery allowed MS patients to regulate their dosage in order to reach an effective (but not psychoactive) level of medication.

GW researchers are now growing strains with varying levels of different cannabinoids, recognizing that each compound has a different effect and that they work best synergistically. It should eventually be possible for the company to market an assortment of different cannabinoid remedies with different concentrations of THC, CBD, and other cannabinoids, terpenes and flavonoids.

Hopefully other innovators will be permitted to pursue similar investigations because a monopoly enforced by prohibition deprives us all of beneficial and effective cannabinoid supplements and treatments.

Heightened Immunity

ROBERT RANDALL EVENTUALLY WITHDREW FROM active involvement with the medical marijuana movement as other players began to take the stage. He was a strong but complicated man, and his role as the founder and guiding light of the movement had given him a sense of responsibility for it. As the AIDS crisis grew, the numbers of patients seeking marijuana vastly increased. The medical marijuana movement was growing beyond Randall's ability to control it, and that frustrated him. For example, he deeply resented and disliked Dennis Peron and his confrontational style of San Francisco activism—despite the fact that it was Peron's daring bravado that re-energized the movement and put marijuana into the pipes of tens of thousands of patients.

Randall had been living secretly with AIDS for years, and in the late 1990s his health began to deteriorate. He attributed his long-term survival without medication to his constant intake of cannabinoids via the NIDA marijuana he still smoked for his glaucoma. Eventually, however, his health failed. Randall died in Florida on June 2, 2001.

Randall's belief that his constant marijuana use extended his survival time and his quality of life may have been correct. At the time, of course, little was known about the broad range of positive health effects that cannabis had and even less about the role played by the endocannabinoid system in achieving those effects. The experience of Randall and other patients was, however, already showing that AIDS patients who used marijuana were tending to live longer and feel better than those who did not.

When Donald Abrams and his research team had successfully completed their Trojan horse study of marijuana's interaction with the protease inhibitor AIDS drugs they found that patients who received cannabinoids—whether in the form of marijuana or dronabinol (Marinol)—had higher CD4 cell counts (a marker of better immune system function) than those who had been given placebos. Even more significantly, they found that those who received marijuana had greater increases in CD8 cells (another marker of immune function) than those who took dronabinol compared to placebo (increases of 20% and 10%, respectively).[151] Cannabinoids also seemed to possess some anti-viral activity.[152] In other words, marijuana is not the immune system destroyer the government had claimed it was—in fact, it actually *improved* the immune system.

> *Marijuana is not the immune system destroyer the government had claimed it was—in fact, it actually improved the immune system.*

The immune-enhancing effects of marijuana were above and beyond what researchers expected. Abrams commented that, "The change in lymphocyte counts for the smoked group is intriguing. At a minimum, it contradicts findings from previous studies suggesting that smoked marijuana suppresses the immune system."[153]

For years, well-funded pseudoscientific studies, such as those conducted and publicized by biased "experts" had claimed that marijuana's "depressant effect on immunity is not a good indication for patients with cancer or AIDS."[154] Abrams' new data, based on an actual clinical trial rather than on animal studies, was exactly what the government did not want to see. Honest research on human subjects proved that the government's propaganda was nothing more than misinformation.

Of course, the data on the immune system and marijuana's interaction with the new HIV drugs had really been a way to get the study approved. The true purpose behind it had been to ascertain whether marijuana helped improve the appetite of AIDS patients—and it did. Both groups of patients who took cannabinoids had significant weight gain. Science had spoken; THC really did cause the munchies.

The success of the Trojan horse study led Abrams to decide to propose a new study, this time to evaluate anecdotal evidence about marijuana's ability to relieve neuropathic pain. Neuropathic pain results from damage to or dysfunction of the peripheral nervous system, and does not respond well to opiate-based drugs. A number of Abrams' own patients were reporting problems with neuropathy as a side-effect of the new HIV drugs.

Unlike the previous study, which had masqueraded as an investigation of the potential harm caused by marijuana, the pain study was explicitly designed to explore its potential benefits. Of course, NIDA had a long history of blocking such research, but times had changed. The power of the CMCR— the new medical cannabis research program funded and supported by the state of California—together with the enormous publicity surrounding the federal research blockade had forced officials to change their behavior. Abrams submitted the protocol for review to the federal government through the CMCR, and for the first time since the development of Dronabinol had ended the state-sponsored cancer studies, NIDA agreed to provide marijuana for a study of its possible benefits for humans. Other CMCR clinical investigators had also begun to secure funding—and marijuana—for research into its positive effects on nausea, sleep, spasticity, and pain associated with cancer.

Unfortunately, a lack of study subjects led to the discontinuation of several CMCR trials, including one of Abrams' own studies designed to assess whether marijuana could help cancer patients reduce the amount of opiate pain killers they were taking. Several reasons have been posited for the lack of cancer patients taking part in medical marijuana research.

One of these is the insistence of the DEA and NIDA that all human marijuana research be conducted at in-patient facilities where subjects are sequestered away from everyone but the research staff. Understandably, many people facing terminal illness would prefer to spend as much of their remaining time as possible with their family and friends, rather than in a hospital.

Another reason cancer patients have been largely unwilling to take part in studies of marijuana has to do with the passage of Proposition 215 and the resulting establishment of a quasi-legitimate medical marijuana industry. The expanded access that patients had to a wide variety of fresh and potent cannabis products also worked to discourage them from signing up for state-sponsored studies. After all, why would a sick patient trade high-quality marijuana from a dispensary for the low-grade product provided by NIDA? It was ironic that the in-patient requirements were intended to prevent subjects from "diverting" their experimental marijuana to their friends. As many patients observed, nobody on the street would want such terrible weed.

NIDA's research requirements presented yet another problem for the recruitment of subjects. NIDA required that all patients go through a "washout period" before the study began, meaning that if they had been using marijuana they would have to go some time without it in order to participate. For people who were using it successfully, this meant a return to suffering—and if they were assigned to a placebo group it would be for the entire duration of the study. For cancer and HIV patients, stopping their marijuana use could have a profoundly negative effect on their long-term health.

After an adjustment period, California's medical marijuana law was largely working although there were instances of law enforcement agents ignoring the law in order to harass and arrest legitimate patients. But the courts were increasingly taking the side of patients. More and more frequently, judges and juries were instructing officials to return seized marijuana to its legal owners. Sometimes, frustrated state police turned the evidence over to DEA officials in an attempt to circumvent state law and send patients to federal prison. Federal agents continued to raid dispensaries and cooperative farms but were less and less able to keep up with their rapid proliferation. It was also getting harder for them to justify their attacks on medical marijuana providers while a real drug epidemic—methamphetamine—was sweeping the nation. Federal drug warriors had realized that they had lost the war for public opinion, and they were becoming desperate. They trotted out the most sensationalistic science they could find on marijuana. They cited bizarre studies making claims such as preteens who smoke five joints a day are a fraction of a percentage more likely to develop mental illness. The public, however, wasn't buying it.

Rather than striving to keep a discredited policy alive with deceit and hysteria, other nations like Canada, Israel, and the Netherlands accepted marijuana's medical value and established pharmaceutical cannabis cultivation and distribution networks. Canada has, for example, been much more receptive to cannabis-based therapies than the U.S. Canadian health regulators established a federal cultivation program to supply patients with marijuana in 2000 and approved GW Pharmaceuticals' Sativex® spray for use by MS patients in 2005. In Israel, Rick Doblin was having a much easier time facilitating research into medical marijuana than he had in the U.S. Clinical trials of marijuana's effectiveness for soldiers suffering from post-traumatic stress disorders were already underway. Israel has always been more receptive to cannabis research, perhaps in part because it is home to the father of cannabis science, Raphael Mechoulam. The Israeli government has been licensing medical cannabis growers since 2008.

> *The change in lymphocyte counts for the smoked group is intriguing. At a minimum, it contradicts findings from previous studies suggesting that smoked marijuana suppresses the immune system.*

In 2002, two of Jeff Jones' Oakland clients, Angel Raich and Diane Monson, brought a case against the DEA, petitioning for access to legal marijuana. Raich was the most extreme example of a desperate patient, as she was suffering from an inoperable brain tumor. Marijuana was the only substance that had worked to help her function in a nearly normal manner. Since she had begun smoking marijuana daily, Raich had been able to get out of her wheelchair and live a relatively normal life. Despite the fact that her case was the clearest example imaginable of a patient in need of medical marijuana, the courts just said "No."

Doctors, too, were taking their case to the courts. Marcus Conant was the lead plaintiff for the group of doctors and patients who sued ONDCP head Gen. Barry McCaffrey, Attorney General Janet Reno, HHS Secretary Donna Shalala, and DEA Administrator Thomas Constantine for threatening to prosecute physicians who recommend medical marijuana to the physicians' patients, thereby violating their Constitutional rights. Conant and company won a unanimous decision from the 9th Circuit Court of Appeals, a decision which the

Supreme Court let stand in October 2003. Following the case, a climate emerged in which some physicians felt free to suggest cannabis to their patients. If their doctors were still wary about the legal and professional ramifications of recommending marijuana, patients could take their paperwork to clinics specializing in providing medical cannabis recommendations.

The Compassionate IND program was established under a federal provision that allowed patients to receive marijuana legally as long as they did so under the auspices of a research program. The patient's physician would (at least in theory) be responsible for gathering information on the drug's effects and side-effects and regularly reporting the data back to the NIH. The program, of course was a ruse—a way to get Robert Randall out of their hair. Federal health authorities didn't really care whether or not they gathered any positive data on marijuana. As DEA Spokesman Don McLearn put it: "There was never any intent of using reports from the Compassionate IND's to reach approval of the drug. In fact, the reports submitted regularly by the participants' doctors are used only to evaluate whether to keep them in the program. The reports have no effect on a policy that discounts the medical value of smoking marijuana." [155]

Others, however, were interested in getting some real data out of the IND program. Ethan Russo, M.D., a neurologist at the University of Montana at Missoula who had been trying unsuccessfully to obtain NIDA cannabis for migraine research, decided that this group was a unique patient population that should be studied. He thought that wasting such valuable data was criminally negligent, and set about making up for lost time.

Four of the seven remaining IND members agreed to take part in an assessment.

The patients, who had been smoking NIDA and/or black market marijuana every day for over 10 years, were tested for both physical and mental health. Russo's conclusions and recommendations were:

- Cannabis smoking, even of a crude low-grade product, provides effective symptomatic relief of pain, muscle spasms, and intraocular pressure elevations in selected patients failing other modes of treatment.

- These clinical cannabis patients are able to reduce or eliminate other prescription medicines and their accompanying side effects.
- Clinical cannabis provides an improved quality of life.
- The side effect profile of NIDA cannabis in chronic usage suggests some mild pulmonary risks.
- No malignant deterioration has been observed.
- No consistent or attributable neuropsychological or neurological deterioration has been observed.
- No endocrine, hematological or immunological sequelae have been observed.
- Improvements in a clinical cannabis program would include a ready and consistent supply of sterilized, potent, organically grown unfertilized female flowering top material, thoroughly cleaned of extraneous, inert fibrous matter.
- It is the authors' opinion that the Compassionate IND program should be reopened and extended to patients in need of clinical cannabis.
- Failing that, local, state and federal laws might be amended to provide regulated and monitored clinical cannabis to suitable candidates.[156]

Once again, a scientific study concluded that even chronic marijuana smoking is both safe and effective. Since these patients were smoking NIDA marijuana—which is inferior in potency and freshness to what is readily available in medical dispensaries—imagine how much better the long-term results would be for someone who smokes or (better yet) vaporizes a smaller quantity of higher quality material. Because of the low potency of the NIDA marijuana, the patients in Russo's study smoked on average more than 10 joints per day, between eight and nine ounces (more than half a pound) per month. Frequency and volume of use had been among the IOM committee's main objections to the smoking of medical marijuana for glaucoma, but Russo's study revealed that their concerns were overblown. Although it works, these glaucoma patients have to smoke consistently throughout the day. In decrying the need to constantly medicate, the committee underestimated the body's ability to handle a consistent supplemental dosage of cannabinoids. Some patients certainly felt that being buzzed was better than going blind, suffering intense pain, or dying. IND glaucoma patient Elvy Musikka, for example, found that she was far more debilitated by the surgeries she had to treat her glaucoma than she was from smoking hourly.

As more states began to introduce medical marijuana bills either via the ballot or through the legislature, Musikka and another IND patient, Irv Rosenfeld, began making regular appearances at public hearings and in the media to testify to the need for patients like them to have a constant supply of marijuana without being considered criminals.

Unlocking The Gateway

CALIFORNIA'S MEDICAL MARIJUANA REVOLUTION WAS roaring across the state. With fewer and fewer hostile and ignorant state legislators, and with physicians free to recommend cannabis to their patients, the climate was extremely conducive to the rise of a veritable medical marijuana industry. Dispensaries were opening in both large and small communities, and suppliers were finding ingenious new ways of delivering cannabinoids to patients. As in the times prior to criminalization, a wide assortment of tinctures, extracts, oral sprays, and balms were now available. Networks of growers and vendors sprang up to move the cannabis from farms and grow rooms to manufacturers, storefronts, and delivery services. Today, almost every sizable community in California has at least one indoor grow shop selling high intensity lights, hydroponic systems, and nutrients. Newspapers, magazines, and catalogues make information about cannabinoid research, dispensary locations, and clone strains as easy to access as the daily news. Many of these publications have achieved high levels of circulation and readership in a time when other print media are waning.

Donald Abrams may be the only researcher who has remained consistently dedicated to studying how inhaled marijuana improves human health. Despite all the political progress, hardly anyone is conducting research into the benefits of whole cannabis for human beings. Because many funders and researcher gatekeepers remain attached to the myth that marijuana is too dangerous to study in people, almost all the research taking place uses synthetic cannabinoids on animals. Abrams' decision to conduct his CMCR study of the Volcano system stemmed in large part from the rise in popularity of vaporizers, but also from the idea that the Volcano was the perfect tool for legitimizing cannabis as a medicine. The IOM panel had explicitly called for more research into alternative delivery devices like the vaporizer, and with its sleek aluminum profile the Volcano looks more like a medical centrifuge device than a bong or pipe.

Abrams had no problem finding recruits for the vaporization study, which was framed as a "proof of concept" pilot study intended to lead to other, larger studies. Eighteen healthy inpatient subjects from 21 to 45 were well compensated for comparing the effects of vaporizing to those of smoking cannabis. The study used NIDA's marijuana cigarettes with potencies of 1.7, 3.4, and 6.8 percent THC. NIDA's marijuana is notoriously old and dry, so the cigarettes were rehydrated overnight in a humidifier. They were each then cut in half, with one portion assigned to be smoked and the other vaporized.

> *Vaporizing instead of smoking also practically eliminated the intake of carbon monoxide and other toxic combustion products.*

The study validated vaporization as a safe and effective delivery method. The researchers learned that while smoking and vaporizing delivered approximately the same amount of THC, absorption of the THC into the body tended to happen faster with the vaporizer. Vaporizing instead of smoking also practically eliminated the intake of carbon monoxide and other toxic combustion products.[157] Once the news got out, the Volcano was quickly embraced by patients and non-patients alike. It has become a regular fixture at cannabis events such as the Cannabis Cup, where one often sees huge, 5-foot long Volcano balloon bags being passed around. Its widespread use, however, has been limited by its high price, with each unit costing between $400 and $500. Users with limited manual dexterity also find it slightly difficult to use, but no more so than rolling a joint.

The growth of the medical marijuana subculture in California has been immensely effective in countering the old reefer madness propaganda. Huge numbers of patients have found marijuana safe and effective for everything from terminal illnesses to anxiety. Drug warriors mock the widespread availability of medical marijuana and accuse many of its users of violating of the intent of the law, but the intent of the law is to protect anyone who uses cannabis medicinally from being arrested—regardless of the illness. Since the scientific evidence overwhelmingly shows that cannabinoids do protect us from a wide range of disease processes, the enthusiastic use of medical marijuana is understandable. It also helps to remember that the constant threat of being arrested and jailed for using marijuana can itself cause intense stress, which promotes mental and physical illness. Avoiding that stress by knowing that one is no longer being treated as a criminal is itself a health benefit.

The DEA and the ONDCP are losing the battle over medical marijuana. Only the diehard prohibitionists still buy their lies and their numbers are shrinking. At the same time, there are more and more voters in favor of medical marijuana. California's Proposition 215 passed with 56 percent of the vote in 1996. In 2004, highly conservative Montana said yes to medical marijuana with 62 percent of the vote. That same year the Vermont legislature passed a bill protecting patients from law enforcement. Rhode Island joined the roster in 2006, New Mexico followed in 2007, then Michigan in 2008 with a stunning 63 percent of the vote. New Jersey passed a bill in 2010 as did the District of Columbia. Arizona's citizens passed their first medical marijuana bill in 1996, but arrogant legislators managed to derail it and subsequent bills until the November, 2010 election when the voters passed a bill that must be implemented. Fourteen other states have legislation pending.

The prohibitionists cling to their tired and irrational ideology but more and more people are learning that "it is a tale told by an idiot, full of sound and fury, Signifying nothing."

Marijuana prohibition is crumbling under the pressure of science. There are now hundreds of dispensaries in California, Colorado and other states that are proof of the viability and respectability of legal marijuana commerce. Physicians are also showing a great deal of support for cannabis: As of 2008, approximately 7,000 U.S. physicians had given medical marijuana authorizations to approximately 400,000 patients.[158]

Some of the most intransigent of institutions are beginning to abandon ideology and alter their perspectives to conform to science. Even the Department of Veterans Affairs has begun allowing patients at its hospitals and clinics to use medical marijuana in states where it is legal. In his book *Marihuana: The Forbidden Medicine*, Lester Grinspoon wrote that, "For more than forty years... the AMA steadfastly maintained a position on marihuana closely allied to that of the Federal Bureau of Narcotics and its successor agencies."[159] Now, this alliance has finally been broken. In November 2009, the American Medical Association's Board of Trustees "urged that marijuana's status as a federal Schedule I controlled substance be reviewed with the goal of facilitating the conduct of clinical research and development of cannabis-based medicines."[160]

> *We believe that an evidence-based review by federal regulatory authorities on the safety and efficacy of marijuana and cannabinoids for therapeutic purposes will likely provide evidence to support both appropriate reclassification and adjustment of federal drug enforcement laws...*

One AMA board member, Edward Langston, M.D., complained, "Despite more than 30 years of clinical research, only a small number of randomized, controlled trials have been conducted on smoked cannabis" and that those studies are "insufficient to satisfy the current standards for a prescription drug product."[161]

The revelatory research into the existence and functions of the endocannabinoid system, along with the vast numbers of patients reporting exceptional effects from cannabis-based remedies, has even forced the most staid of physicians' groups to reevaluate their positions on marijuana. One of these, the prestigious American College of Physicians, called for a scientific review of marijuana's classificatory status. "We believe that an evidence-based review by federal regulatory authorities on the safety and efficacy of marijuana and cannabinoids for therapeutic purposes will likely provide evidence to support both appropriate reclassification and adjustment of federal drug enforcement laws..."[162]

Just days after the passage of Proposition 215, Dennis Peron was quoted in *The New York Times* saying that "all use is medical use." Many who had worked on the campaign cringed. It was felt that his comments were deeply irresponsible and that such claims had the potential to sabotage the efforts to help those who were actually ill.

"Why do people smoke pot?" Peron asked when I confronted him about the validity of the statement. "To feel good. That's medical use."

Most supporters of the new law felt that his comment was flippant, and it was, yet, there was also a sense in which Peron was correct. Scientists now have a much better grasp of how cannabinoids act in our bodies. We know that it is not just about feeling good, but also about maintaining physical and mental health. Marijuana's ability to protect us from cancer, Alzheimer's disease, and brain damage means that even recreational use has profoundly healthful side-effects. The rising tide of scientific evidence will continue to erode away the foundations of the war on marijuana, because marijuana really is a gateway to health.

THE SON OF REEFER MADNESS

AS SCIENCE CONFIRMS THAT MARIJUANA is a beneficial herb and not the poisonous weed that ideologues accuse it of being, its opponents grasp ever more desperately to find ways to justify its continued criminalization. They assiduously search for some anecdote or piece of pseudoscientific data to persuade the public—which is becoming increasingly intolerant of their claims—that we must continue throwing users, growers, and vendors of marijuana in prison and prevent the ill from accessing it. Despite the fact that most justifications for criminalizing marijuana have been refuted by peer-reviewed clinical research, prohibitionists still promulgate fallacies as fact. Take, for example, NIDA's claim on its Web site that long-term marijuana use "increases risk of cancer of the head, neck, and lungs."[163]

This is the complete opposite of the truth. Such blatant lies are particularly insidious because they serve to discourage people from taking part in an activity that actually decreases the likelihood of developing cancer. The evidence, as we have seen, is clear and undeniable: marijuana protects users from developing lung and head and neck cancers. So despite the fact that we have had solid evidence of marijuana's anticarcinogenic properties since 1975, government agencies continue to use taxpayers' money to lie to them.

Another claim NIDA has made about marijuana is that it "increases the risk of chronic cough, bronchitis and emphysema."[164] This statement is deliberately misleading. It is true that regularly smoking harsh marijuana using certain methods can cause chronic cough and bronchitis. Marijuana that is old and dry with low potency (such as the type that NIDA provides to researchers), smoked through a short-stemmed pipe or a joint—which delivers hot smoke directly into the lungs—is most likely to do so. More potent marijuana, however, when smoked through a carbureted pipe (which mixes the smoke with air), a water pipe (which filters and cools it through water), or vaporized (which produces no smoke at all), is much less likely to cause upper respiratory irritation.

It is completely incorrect, however, to claim that marijuana causes emphysema. Emphysema, also known as chronic obstructive pulmonary disease (COPD), involves the constriction of airways resulting in impaired delivery of oxygen to the blood. It is the fourth leading cause of death in the U.S., and is most often caused by (legal) tobacco

I was amazed that after smoking marijuana the airways actually opened up—dilated—in contrast to the effect of tobacco, Tashkin stated.

smoking. As Donald Tashkin, a leading researcher of marijuana's effect on lung function, has discovered, marijuana smoking is not associated with declines in lung function over time. "I was amazed that after smoking marijuana the airways actually opened up—dilated—in contrast to the effect of tobacco," Tashkin stated.[165]

The NIDA web site also claims that marijuana "impairs coordination and balance."[166] Once again, the actual evidence points to the contrary. A study conducted at the University of Missouri actually found that "marijuana use may be associated with a decreased risk of injury."[167]

Data from a Swiss hospital provides support for these results, even going a step further to suggest that "relative risks decreased with increasing levels of use."[168] In other words, the more you smoke, the less likely you are to have an accident or injury. To claim that marijuana users have fewer accidents than nonusers may seem strange, but remember that the clinical trials of rimonabant reported a negative relationship between cannabinoids and motor impairment. In those studies, patients taking rimonabant—which blocks the action of cannabinoids—experienced more dizziness, vertigo, motor impairment, and cognitive difficulties than those who only took a placebo.[169] As the FDA committee that reviewed the study noted, these effects may well have been the reason why many of the subjects sustained injuries (including contusions, concussions, falls, traffic accidents, and whiplash) during the study.[170] It is quite possible that proper nourishment of the endocannabinoid system helps to activate the brain regions involved in cognitive and motor coordination. Does this mean that accident-prone people could benefit from using marijuana? The evidence seems to suggest just that.

NIDA's claim that marijuana "impairs short-term memory" deserves some discussion.[171] In fact, it may be somewhat correct, though it is probably more accurate to state that marijuana *alters* short-term memory (in part because the word "impairs" suggests physical damage, which is not occurring). According to Italian researcher Vicenzo Di Marzo, the endocannabinoid system accomplishes five things: relaxation, eating, sleeping, protection, and forgetting. Raphael Mechoulam thinks that forgetting might not actually be a bad thing. "Don't think forgetting is less important than recalling," he writes in an

> *There were no significant differences in cognitive decline between heavy users, light users, and nonusers of cannabis.*

article on endocannabinoids. "We should have a system to forget, otherwise... we can burst. If you go down a mall and see a thousand faces do you want to remember all of them? Of course not."[172]

What could be the benefit of temporarily reduced short-term memory? When using marijuana, the ordinary becomes extraordinary. Perhaps marijuana's most enjoyable quality is its ability to alleviate the sense of the mundane—things that one sees, hears, tastes, or thinks everyday shine with qualities that were previously overlooked. Music that one has heard repeatedly suddenly sounds new, full of wonder and emotion. Simple foods can taste like gourmet cuisine.

With the mind liberated from mundane thought patterns, new ideas and insights emerge into consciousness. This can enhance creative expression while temporarily compromising short-term memory. The impact of marijuana use on creativity has not been ignored. Filmmaker Kevin Smith credits marijuana smoking with helping him to get out of a creative slump. He has proclaimed that marijuana "takes me places,

[on] magical journeys. I swear I've never done more writing than when I've been smoking weed for the last six months." [173]

Nevertheless, it is true that the euphoria induced by marijuana can be distracting and potentially inconvenient if one is not careful. You might, for example, forget where you placed your keys, but this is something to be aware of before you indulge. Novice marijuana users are certainly more likely to experience disorientation than regular users, who develop a partial tolerance and who learn to compensate for its effects—like instinctively checking for keys, wallet, and cell phone after using it. It is also worth suggesting that long-term marijuana smokers may actually have fewer forgetful incidents than nonsmokers. Chronic marijuana use increases neurogenesis in adults, thus reducing the chances of developing Alzheimer's and other diseases of cognition and memory. If I had to choose between having to occasionally search for my keys now or forgetting what keys are used for when I'm older, the choice is easy. Another example of the type of short term memory loss associated with using marijuana is losing one's train of thought mid-sentence. Forgetting what you are saying is not due to some toxic insult to the central nervous system, but rather about distraction. It may be hard to keep track of your thoughts when you're enraptured by wonder and sensation. This explains why it is probably not a good idea to get high before going to class or receiving on-the-job training—unless, of course, it's an art or music class.

Nonetheless, there is no credible evidence that long-term marijuana use interferes with memory. An examination of memory following 12 years of cannabis use in individuals under the age of 65 determined that, "There were no significant differences in cognitive decline between heavy users, light users, and nonusers of cannabis." [174]

Another group of researchers found that "compared with placebo, neither marijuana nor dronabinol significantly altered performance on any of the [cognitive function] tasks." [175]

Disinformation is generated to fuel scare campaigns by pseudoscience research like the study at the Center for Molecular and Behavioral Neuroscience at Rutgers that found that rats injected with a synthetic cannabinoid have memory impairment. This data is now being used as evidence that marijuana permanently damages the brain's ability to retain memories. Other studies have injected rats with pure THC and found that they had a tough time negotiating a maze. These so-called studies are dishonest and wasteful expenditures of taxpayer dollars and have no real-world applications. No one is mainlining marijuana, THC or artificial cannabinoids.

Another piece of hype that NIDA and drug warriors like to circulate is marijuana's potential for addiction. This is simply nonsense: Marijuana is not addictive in the way that heroin, cocaine, methamphetamine, caffeine, and alcohol are. This is not to say that a small percentage of marijuana users have not developed problematic relationships with it, but these are few and far between especially when compared to the degenerative misery that is alcoholism. I will address problematic marijuana usage in greater detail in a later chapter.

Because of its pleasurable effects, many of those committed to demonizing marijuana try to label all use as addiction or abuse. Scientific research confirms that the euphoria that many people experience when using marijuana is not the result of a toxic insult to the central nervous system (as with alcohol) but rather yet another aspect of its healthful

> *Compared with placebo, neither marijuana nor dronabinol significantly altered performance on any of the [cognitive function] tasks.*

effects. Just as the sweetness of the mango induces us to eat its vitamin and mineral-rich flesh, the pleasure of using marijuana encourages us to ingest its cancer-inhibiting and life-improving cannabinoids.

While it is impossible to die of a marijuana overdose, it is possible to use too much. Anything taken to its extreme will manifest its opposite: Too much mango gives you a stomach ache and runny stool, and too much marijuana can make you uncomfortable, dizzy, and possibly even a little nauseated.

Unless handled improperly, however, this situation is not health-threatening. "Psychological overdoses" happen most often with marijuana edibles; the primary reason for this is that many people view eating marijuana as somehow being more benign and innocent than smoking it. They reason that while smoking is a vice, everyone eats.

Smoked or vaporized cannabinoids enter the blood stream immediately and are quickly relayed to the brain. Because of the long time it takes to digest food, however, it is almost impossible to estimate a dosage effectively when eating or drinking products containing marijuana. When eaten, cannabinoids must go through the digestive process before they are delivered to the bloodstream. They must then pass through the liver, which not only takes more time but also converts one cannabinoid into a more potent form that produces a much "heavier" high. A marijuana cupcake might seem cute and innocent, but it can pack a much stronger punch than a few puffs from a bong or joint.

Sometimes the results of such confusion can be comical. Consider the transcript of a 911 call from one Officer Sanchez, who discovered this possibility when he baked some brownies using confiscated marijuana.

Sanchez: Can you please send rescue? I think I'm having an overdose and so is my wife.

911: Overdose of what?

Sanchez: Marijuana. I don't know if it had something in it.

911: OK.

Sanchez: Can you please send rescue?

911: OK, how old are you?

Sanchez: I'm 28, uhh, 29-years-old, and my wife is 26. Please come.

911: Have you guys been drinking also?

Sanchez: No, that's it.

911: Is there any weapons in the house?

Sanchez: No. Please come!

911: Do you guys have fever or anything?

Sanchez: No. I think we're dying.

911: How much did you guys have?

Sanchez: I don't know. We made brownies and I think we're dead. I really do.

911: OK. How much did you put in the brownies? Was it a bag? Who made the brownies?

Sanchez: My wife and I did.

911: OK, get her.

Sanchez: She's on the living room ground right now.

911: Is she breathing?

Sanchez: She's barely breathing.

911: Is she awake?

Sanchez: I think so.

911: Can you look?

Sanchez: Yeah, I can feel her she's laying down right in front of me. Time is going by really, really, really slow.[176]

It should come as no surprise to learn that Officer Sanchez had to resign from the police department after his marijuana misadventure. To call 911 in cases of marijuana overdose is a waste of resources that responders might need to handle a real medical emergency. Instead of panicking, one should relax, breath deeply, put on some favorite music, or even sing. Philosopher and explorer Terence McKenna once suggested singing "Row Row Row Your Boat" if one is having a difficult time involving an altered state of consciousness. "It gets air into your lungs and once you reach the part about 'life is but a dream' the metaphysical implications of that will send you down a whole new path of thinking," he advised.

The best thing to do in such cases may be to eat something and (unless one is too incapacitated) take a hot shower. Drink water and think of pleasant things. Try watching a slapstick comedy, but avoid the news. No matter how high you get, as long as you stay on the couch you will not do yourself any serious harm. It may even help to tell yourself that at least you're protecting yourself from cancer and brain damage. The worst of the high is over in about two or three hours, though it could seem like two or three days. Even veteran cannabis users should start slowly with edibles. Unless you know the potency, it is always better to start with half or a quarter of the full dose. Legalization will help reduce the frequency of such unpleasant experiences, since marijuana products will be produced with known and uniform doses of cannabinoids.

In the meantime, opponents of marijuana use will say anything to frighten people away from it. Among their spurious claims is the absurd assertion that "marijuana today is a very different plant from that of yesterday." The truth is that it is actually still just cannabis. Growing conditions have been optimized and growth cycles have been manipulated in order to maximize potency and increase the number of harvests, but it is the same plant. The "new marijuana" disinformation campaign wants to make it seem like the cannabis of today has been genetically engineered into something more like heroin or PCP than marijuana.

That said, it is true that due to advances in outdoor and indoor growing techniques, potent marijuana is more available now than it was in the 1970s and 1980s. There was some very strong marijuana in those years; it was just harder to obtain. Connoisseurs sought out potent strains like Maui Wowie, Big Sur Holy Weed, Panama Red, and Ice Bag. Keith Stroup, the founder of NORML, dismisses the "new marijuana" campaign: "We got plenty high back then."

In fact, stronger marijuana is actually better for you. A higher ratio of cannabinoids to plant material means that the same effects are achieved while less volume is smoked. Potent marijuana gives you more tumor-fighting compounds and fewer harmful combustion by-products. So if you haven't smoked much marijuana since the 1970s or early 1980s, start slowly. Whereas before you might have needed an entire joint, today one or two puffs could suffice. So once again, claims about the "new marijuana" are entirely overblown. While it is much easier to access high-quality marijuana than it used to be, it is still the same plant and it is still not dangerous.

The "new marijuana" scare campaign was devised as a way to persuade Baby Boomers not to dismiss their teenage children's experimentation with marijuana as the same harmless rite of passage that they experienced in the 1970s. The prohibitionists correctly identified that a huge population of former and current marijuana smokers who had started in their teens and survived and thrived would be unalarmed with their own teenagers trying it out. In fact, many preferred that their kids use marijuana in lieu of alcohol. In order to coax these boomers aboard the reefer madness express, the federal anti-drug agencies created the myth of the "new marijuana." They took the kernel of truth that strong marijuana was more available, and spun it into a tale of "New Marijuana" and "Deadly Dope."

Here is an example of the sensational propaganda from HHS's Substance Abuse and Mental Health Services Administration: "Even though you or your friends might have smoked pot when you were younger, your teen should steer clear of marijuana. It's much stronger today than it was decades ago. Some reports estimate that today's marijuana is five times the strength than it was in the 1970s, while other reports estimate the strength to be 25 times that of earlier decades. Basically, it's a totally different drug."[177]

This is your government lying to you. First, the statistics that the feds use to arrive at these values are manipulated to the point of torture.

They take the potency values for the entire amount of seized cannabis from the 1970s and then cook them down into an average. There are two considerations when looking at these artificially low values. First, the government was seizing a lot of feral hemp from the Midwest, low-THC fiber hemp plants escaped from the Hemp for Victory farming campaign in the 1940s, better known as "ditch weed." These plants, having 1% or less THC, diluted the potency pool as they were seized and burned by the ton. Secondly, the instrumentation used to measure THC levels in the 1970s and early 1980s was comparatively primitive and inefficient by today's standards. The average potency of marijuana smoked in the 1970s probably ran to around 4 to 8 percent THC, some was very strong, most was strong enough and some was weak—but still active.

According to data from NIDA, the average THC content during 2008 was 10.1%. If you accept SAMHSA's claim of a five-fold increase in potency and divide this value by 5, you get 2% THC. And 10.1% divided by 25 gives you .25% THC which was never going to sell to any repeat customers. What the federal deceivers have done is to take the lowest average potency values from three decades ago and compare them to recent specific individual samples of optimally potent marijuana. Once again, the "new marijuana" is the same plant grown in optimal conditions and harvested at the perfect peak of potency. And if, as the marijuana opponents assert, cannabis lovers have been able to take a plant and increase its yield to 25 times what it was before they began working with it, well this should nullify any claims that stoners are amotivated underachievers. The alarmists also conveniently ignore the fact that in much of the world, cannabis is consumed and has been consumed for thousands of years, not as marijuana, but as hashish which is the gathered and pressed resin glands from the cannabis buds. Since making hashish concentrates the most potent part of the plant into a resin lump or ball, it is far more powerful than even the strongest marijuana and has been used for thousands of years without serious concerns.

At Harborside Health Center, in Oakland, California, strains of marijuana are labeled with their potency and cannabinoid content so that patients can choose the appropriate one for their needs. Knowing the cannabinoid content of the marijuana allows people to adjust their intake more effectively to reach the desired results. A number of other dispensaries are now following Harborside's lead in offering marijuana that has been analyzed for potency and purity. Other analytical labs, such as Montana Botanical Analysis, CannabAnalysis Laboratories and Botanical Analytics are springing up in states where medical cannabis is allowed. Since drug warriors are so concerned about the increased availability of high-quality marijuana, the best response would be to legalize cannabis cultivation, thus allowing patients and consumers to know what they are getting in order to select less powerful strains.

The "new marijuana" campaign has become just one part of a much broader propaganda push, which we could call the "new reefer madness." The myth of the "new marijuana" serves as a springboard for opponents of marijuana to launch even more hysterical attacks on its effects. Among these attacks, the most prominent is aimed at convincing the public that marijuana, especially the "new marijuana," causes schizophrenia and mental illness in teenagers, and that it is therefore too dangerous to legalize or decriminalize.

This new disinformation campaign began around the time that the medical marijuana movement was gaining strength. The foundation of the new hysteria was a poorly-conducted study of cannabis and schizophrenia in Swedish military conscripts—certainly a rather rarified population. The study found that regular cannabis users were six times more likely to develop schizophrenia than non-users.[178]

In their 1997 book, *Marijuana Myths/Marijuana Facts,* Lynn Zimmer, Ph.D. and John Morgan, M.D., examined the Swedish study and concluded:

> Heavy cannabis use was only one of many factors present at age eighteen that was associated with a later diagnosis of schizophrenia. In fact, all of the later schizophrenics had been given a psychiatric diagnosis of some sort by military psychiatrists at the point of conscription. All had been prescribed medication for "nervous problems." All had come from broken homes and all had, at some point in their lives, been in trouble at school and in trouble with the police. In other words, in this sample, heavy cannabis use was associated with a variety of psychological and social problems, all of which were also associated with a later diagnosis of schizophrenia.[179]

Because the bulk of the marijuana research funded by the vast wealth of the federal government is intended to assess harm, ideologically and financially-driven researchers will deliberately craft studies to get the desired results (i.e., evidence of harm) in order to obtain additional funding.

Sometimes, of course, such studies produce anomalous results. One of these was the National Toxicology Project trial in which rats and mice were given large doses of THC. Rather than finding evidence of harm, researchers instead discovered that the more THC the rodents received, the fewer tumors they had and the longer they lived.(see Chapter 2) The Swedish study, however, found just what it was looking for—albeit with questionable methods. As a result, its publication encouraged many researchers to design studies specifically to confirm that marijuana poses a severe threat to mental health.

The renewed movement to associate marijuana use with mental illness was first initiated in Great Britain, following the country's reclassification of cannabis from a Class B to a Class C substance (which reduced the punishment for possession from arrest to a warning). Prohibitionists on both sides of the political spectrum trumpeted the results of questionable surveys as proof that the "new marijuana," called "skunk" in Britain, is a mind-destroying poison that must be more heavily criminalized.

In 2005, U.K. Home Secretary Jacqui Smith asked the Advisory Council on the Misuse of Drugs to reverse marijuana's reclassification but the Council advised keeping it in Class C. In 2007, Smith again requested a review of marijuana's classification because of the threat of skunk. Following an exhaustive review by almost 30 researchers, the Council again determined that cannabis products should remain in Class C.

Smith's successor Alan Johnson and Prime Minister Gordon Brown were undeterred by the Council's recommendations and began pushing to re-criminalize marijuana. Brown, fancying himself quite the science expert, said, "I don't think that the previous studies took into account that so much of the cannabis on the streets is now of a lethal quality and we really have got to send out a message to young people—this is not acceptable."[180] The nation's chief drug advisor, David Nutt, M.D., protested the push to move cannabis back to Class B. After insisting that marijuana, LSD, and Ecstasy were much less harmful than alcohol, he was fired from the Advisory Council. This Nixonian move turned out to be ill-advised when it backfired, generating enormous sympathetic publicity for Nutt and providing him with huge amounts of media time to make his case and condemn the politicians.

"Do not ask scientists to produce evidence to justify a moral stance," Nutt protested. "If you don't like what we say about the science then say, 'Okay, we'll take a moral position,' but don't try to tell me the science we've done is wrong!"[181]

Like Nutt, a number of other Council members were appalled at the intrusion of politics into the sanctity of the research laboratory. Many of them resigned in protest. Other scientists uninvolved with drug regulation also pointed out that to sabotage science so blatantly would cast doubt on all of the government's decisions—in the eyes of the public as well as the researchers.

Nutt and a diverse group of pharmacologists, toxicologists, and epidemiologists responded to the Home Secretary's "appalling contempt for science" by establishing a new independent scientific review body, the Independent Scientific Committee on Drugs, to determine the risks and benefits of legal and illegal psychoactive substances without the taint of political pressure.

Nonetheless, the hysterical skunk and schizophrenia campaign in the U.K. did succeed in pushing marijuana back into Schedule B. Seeing how successful it was in the U.K., drug warriors in the U.S. decided to seize upon the propaganda in a failed attempt to derail the medical marijuana movement.

Smoking marijuana is a relatively new phenomenon in Great Britain. Prior to the 1990s, concentrated cannabis in the form of hashish or resin was more frequently used than the dried material of the plant. Despite the fact that hashish is more potent than "Skunk," the novelty of smoking the actual plant matter enabled propagandists to convince the public that it was a dangerous trend. By contrast, marijuana has been the main cannabis product in the U.S. since the 1930s and hashish was much less common. This meant that it was not as easy to startle the American public by convincing them that the marijuana they or their friends had smoked was dangerous enough to transform its users into psychotic menaces.

When we ignore studies specifically designed to show evidence of harm and look instead at the true science concerning marijuana and schizophrenia, what do we find? Lester Grinspoon, an expert in both fields and the co-author of *Schizophrenia: Pharmacotherapy and Psychotherapy* and other textbooks thinks the answer is clear. "It's hard to refute a study that says certain things are going to happen in the years ahead, but smoking marijuana does not *cause* schizophrenia."[182] Grinspoon explains that there is not "even a blip in the incidence of schizophrenia in the U.S. after millions of people started smoking marijuana in the 1960s."[183]

The British medical journal *The Lancet* published a meta-analysis of the relevant data and reached similar conclusions. "If the relation between [cannabis] use and schizophrenia were truly causal and if the relative risk was around five-fold, then the incidence of schizophrenia should have more than doubled since 1970. However, population trends in schizophrenia incidence suggest that incidence has either been stable or slightly decreased over the relevant period of time."[184]

> *Smoking marijuana does not cause schizophrenia.*

Colin Blakemore, Ph.D., of the University of Oxford is slightly more cautious, but agrees that links between cannabis and schizophrenia are tenuous at best.

> It is conceivable that the excessive use of cannabis sometimes contributes to acute schizophrenic episodes. But it is difficult to believe that cannabis is a strong risk factor for this disorder, because there is no evidence that the incidence of schizophrenia has risen dramatically over the past 50 years, in parallel with the huge increase in cannabis use. Young schizophrenic patients are often heavy cigarette smokers too, but no-one would suggest that tobacco causes schizophrenia.[185]

Also, research scientists at Keele University in the U.K. conducted a study of over half a million patients between 1996 and 2005, and determined that "the causal models linking cannabis with schizophrenia/psychoses are not supported" and that, despite the rapid rise in cannabis use, the rate of schizophrenia and psychoses remained stable or even declined over the period of the study.[186]

According to some experts, the true link between schizophrenia and cannabis use is one of self-medication. Many young people with a tendency to develop the disease find that smoking marijuana eases their symptoms and they pursue its use, perhaps lacking the judgment necessary to adequately titrate their dosage. Given marijuana's ability to protect the brain and induce neurogenesis, it is highly unlikely that using it would induce the type of damage associated with schizophrenia—and highly likely that those with the disease would seek it out for those helpful effects. When cannabis is once again legal, it will be much easier to determine what ratio of cannabinoids these patients need to optimize their mental health and how to deliver it to them appropriately.

There seems to be a good deal of support for the idea that those with a tendency toward schizophrenia may use marijuana to treat their symptoms. For example, a study using pure THC (which is far stronger than the most potent "new marijuana" or skunk) found that patients with severe chronic schizophrenia who admitted to self-medicating with marijuana improved after using the drug. The researchers concluded that such data could "open a possible new role for cannabinoids in the treatment of schizophrenia." [187] Another study found that the cannabinoid CBD was associated with significant decreases in psychotic symptoms and had fewer side-effects than amisulpride, a commonly used antipsychotic drug. [188] Studies like these highlight once again the importance of legalization, which will allow for the development of cannabinoid-based remedies with specific formulations for specific illnesses. Since THC and CBD have both been shown to have antipsychotic properties, it is likely that they work together in what Raphael Mechoulam calls the "entourage effect." While they work well on their own, their benefits for mental health are even greater when used in combination. As we move towards legalization, and consequently have greater access to a broad variety of marijuana strains, it is possible that we will see a drop in the incidence of schizophrenia.

To better understand how pseudoscience is geared to produce results "proving" marijuana to be harmful and dangerous, consider a 2009 study that is a shining example of how "experts" generate clinical misinformation. Despite what we now understand about the ability of cannabinoids to protect the lungs from cancer and COPD, this group of researchers claimed that "marijuana smoke caused significantly more damage to cells and DNA than tobacco smoke." [189]

What a frightening claim: Marijuana is more damaging to cells than tobacco. How did scientists generate data that is so contradictory to the vast majority of clinical and epidemiological evidence?

One look at their methods reveals what happened. According to the researchers, they "exposed cultured animal cells and bacteria to condensed smoke samples from both tobacco and marijuana."[190]

In other words, the researchers took cells from (nonhuman) animals and bacteria, multiplied them in Petri dishes, essentially suffocated them with marijuana and tobacco smoke, and compared the results. This is hardly a real-world model: This is very different from what happens when human cells in the body are exposed to marijuana and tobacco.

A tremendous amount of money has been wasted trying to generate reefer madness cloaked as science in order to preserve and perpetuate unjust laws. Yet another ideologically-driven study was conducted in New Zealand, and was released shortly after Donald Tashkin's study of marijuana and lung cancer at UCLA. In direct contradiction to Tashkin's findings, the authors claimed that marijuana use was actually more dangerous than tobacco when it came to developing lung cancer. The gullible media blared out headlines such as "Lung Cancer Risk of One Marijuana Joint a Day Equals a Pack of Cigarettes" without considering the absolute absurdity of the claim.

The conclusions of this "study" are at odds with nearly all other evidence available on marijuana and lung cancer. Understandably, Tashkin—a NIDA scientist whose honesty overcame his prohibitionist leanings—found them extremely puzzling. When he examined the methodology and data, he charged the New Zealand researchers with deliberately misleading the public.

> "There is some cognitive dissonance associated with the findings from this study, at least the interpretation of the findings, and I think that has to do with the belief model among the investigators and I hate to say it—they're not here to defend themselves—but with the integrity of the investigators. So what they did was a statistical sleight of hand. They are implying that smokers of only 365 joints of marijuana have a risk of developing lung cancer that is similar to that of 7000 tobacco cigarettes, something that is just, as I said, an excellent example of cognitive dissonance."[191]

When we hear sensational news reports about the dangers of using marijuana, it helps to be suspicious. There is simply no honest data suggesting any harm associated with even heavy, long-term, regular use of marijuana—other than bronchitis for those who use harsh material without cooling the smoke. Nearly, all of the scientific data concerning marijuana's effects point to benefits for the user. Tragically, all too often the scientifically illiterate media regurgitates the results of dishonest studies without examining the methodology, and then dresses them up with an extra layer of hysteria.

A headline appearing in December 2009 is an excellent illustration of this type of media-fueled debacle. When a study associating cannabis use and brain damage in youth appeared, the news media wallowed in the same type of reefer madness that Anslinger employed in the 1930s. *ScienceDaily.com* introduced the story with the tabloid headline, "Cannabis Damages Young Brains More Than Originally Thought, Study Finds" and warned of "an irreversible, long-term effect on the brain." [192]

Canadian website *Healthzone* also ventured into yellow journalism with the headline, "Cannabis brain damage worse in teens than thought." [193] The story was illustrated with a photo of a young woman smoking an enormous, flaming joint that looked more like the Olympic torch than a standard marijuana cigarette.

Emaxhealth.com parroted that "cannabis [is] more damaging to adolescent brains than previously known," and falsely claimed that "the study is the first to focus on long-term effects of cannabis use among teens." [194] As it turns out, the study had nothing whatsoever to do with cannabis use among teenagers. The study had actually looked at what happened to adolescent rats after being heavily dosed with a synthetic cannabinoid that was far more potent than THC. Nothing about the study resembled the real-world use of marijuana by adolescent human beings, and despite this the pitifully ignorant and/or complicit media treated it as a profound scientific revelation.

(It is worth noting that there are a number of reasons having nothing to do with brain damage that adolescents should not regularly use marijuana. I will address this more in the next chapter.)

Because it oversees about 85 percent of the world's research into controlled substances, NIDA's monopoly on marijuana and cannabinoid research directly affects the state of global health. The blockade that it maintains on research into marijuana's positive health effects continues to thwart the development of new preventatives and treatments for cancer, Alzheimer's and other diseases. Sometimes, NIDA makes an active effort to hide the fact that marijuana fights cancer and stimulates neurogenesis. The agency has claimed that "THC overstimulates the cannabinoid receptors, leading to a disruption of the endogenous cannabinoids' normal function."[195] The implication is that "disruption" is undesirable—but if "normal function" means getting cancer and Alzheimer's, isn't disruption a good thing?

NIDA spokesperson Shirley Simson once again reminds us, "As the National Institute on Drug Abuse, our focus is primarily on the negative consequences of marijuana use. We generally do not fund research focused on the potential beneficial medical effects of marijuana."[196]

So, who does? Hardly anyone since the closing of the CMCR due to California's state budget crisis. Even the more basic research that NIDA funds into the activity of cannabinoids and cannabinoid receptors is primarily conducted with synthetic cannabinoids, which (as they well know) makes generalizing its results to herbal cannabis extremely difficult. By restricting research to synthetic cannabinoids, ideologues are able to falsely claim that natural molecules will somehow overload and damage the cannabinoid receptors.

These claims are deceptions built on distortions of science. There is no reason to believe that synthetic THC is safer or more effective than the naturally-occurring version. In fact, there are serious reasons to believe just the opposite.

For instance, a study comparing the effects of marijuana and synthetic THC in AIDS patients determined that both "dronabinol and marijuana produce comparable increases in food intake and improve mood without producing disruptions in psychomotor functioning." Marijuana, however, had the added benefit of improving sleep.[197] Because the science of cannabis has been hobbled by anti-marijuana hysteria for so many years, we remain largely ignorant of the therapeutic potential of most cannabinoids and of how they work together in the entourage effect. Hopefully, the public will begin demanding even more vocally that the legal restrictions on marijuana be lifted so that an entirely new field and industry of cannabinoid supplements and remedies can arise.

The exploration, development, and use of synthetic cannabinoids should also continue so long as it does not stand in the way of research into phytocannabinoids.

Although many of the studies cited in this book were conducted with synthetic cannabinoids, epidemiological studies nevertheless suggest that many of the results could also be applicable to phytocannabinoids. Natural cannabis products with a diverse range of cannabinoid ratios need to be investigated if appropriate therapeutic applications are to be developed—especially considering research that has shown that marijuana's ability to inhibit brain cancer has to do with the way THC and CBD work together.[198] When prohibition ends, research into targeted cannabinoid applications, and possible cocktails with conventional treatments, could progress rapidly and expand on the model set by GW Pharmaceuticals.

The federal government continues to stand in the way of medical marijuana research. In January 2010, despite the Obama Administration's directive to the DEA to honor state medical marijuana laws, the DEA raided Full Spectrum Laboratories, a Colorado facility that was assessing the composition, potency, and safety of medical marijuana. Consequently, Colorado's patients trying to find the proper strain of medicine for their needs were once again consigned to trial and error.

Even those who decide to navigate the bureaucratic nightmare of federal licensing are repeatedly thwarted. Lyle Craker, Professor of Plant and Soil Sciences at the University of Massachusetts, has for years been trying to get a license to cultivate medical-grade cannabis plants for research. The DEA has continuously blocked his efforts, acting as an institutional henchman to preserve NIDA's monopoly on research marijuana. The entanglement of NIDA and the DEA in a kind of institutional incest works against the best interests of the American people by preventing the development of much-needed medicines.

Opponents of medical marijuana and legalization have a number of theories that they like to use to convince people of the harms of marijuana. Among these is the gateway theory: the claim that there is something about marijuana that makes its users more likely to "graduate" to harder drugs, like cocaine and heroin. Contrary to what drug warriors would have you believe, the gateway theory could not be farther from the truth. In fact, it can be dispelled with simple-minded observation: Statistics show that over 40 percent of Americans have ever used marijuana while only 1.3 percent have used heroin. That's a pretty poor conversion rate for a gateway drug.

Marijuana is not a gateway to other drugs; it is a gateway to health. In fact, it could actually help people overcome addictions to more dangerous drugs, such as alcohol. Film director Robert Altman was among those for whom marijuana was a gateway to health. "I was a heavy drinker, but alcohol affected my heart rather than my liver. So I stopped," Altman remembered in 1992. "And I miss it. I really like that kind of life. I smoke grass now. I say that to everybody, because marijuana should be legalized. It's ridiculous that it isn't." Another person whose switch from alcohol to marijuana saved his health is the fine arts patron and billionaire Peter Lewis, who helped fund the passage of California's Proposition 215. "Marijuana is, for almost everybody who uses it, a positive. It improves the quality of life, it improves performance. It improves."

> *Statistics show that over 40 percent of Americans have ever used marijuana while only 1.3 percent have used heroin. That's a pretty poor conversion rate for a gateway drug.*

If there is any association between marijuana and other drugs it is the direct result of its criminal status. According to the government, marijuana and heroin have the same potential for abuse and the same lack of medical uses. When federal authorities send the message that marijuana and heroin are equally dangerous, naïve users are bound to get into trouble. When young people who try marijuana find that it is not the deadly poison they were told it was, and they see heroin on the same list, what are they to think? Many of them are not sophisticated enough to know that while marijuana is a completely nontoxic substance, heroin can suppress the areas of the brain that control breathing—sometimes with deadly results. Many of them have also not been told that, unlike the mild dependence that a small percentage of heavy marijuana users experience, heroin addiction is real and tenacious. Scheduling marijuana and much more dangerous drugs in the same category is bureaucratic immorality.

Research confirms that the gateway theory of marijuana is a myth. The Institute of Medicine report, to cite one powerful example, pointed out that there is a big difference between claiming users of heavier drugs tend to start with marijuana and claiming that marijuana actually led them on to heavier drugs.

Because marijuana use typically precedes rather than follows initiation into the use of other illicit drugs, it is assailed as being a gateway drug. However it does not appear to be a gateway drug to the extent that it is the cause or even that it is the most significant predictor of serious drug abuse; that is *care must be taken not to attribute cause to association.*[199] Experimental research on animals, while not directly generalizable to humans, also suggests that marijuana does not lead automatically to more dangerous drugs. "Marijuana does not prime animals to self-administer heroin or cocaine in experimental addiction research."[200] So much for the gateway drug theory.

Many opponents of marijuana also cite concerns about driving. If marijuana is legalized, how would we address the issue of driving while high? Compared to alcohol drinkers, marijuana smokers have a stronger sense of self-preservation. Marijuana does not slay good judgment in the way that alcohol does. Whereas marijuana tends to increase cautious behaviors, alcohol obliterates the sense of safety and sensibility. Most of us are familiar with the drunken fool belligerently insisting that he's capable of driving himself home. The good thing about marijuana and driving is that you tend to know when you're too high to drive. Instead of drunken delusional bravado, there is a slight horror at the very idea of having to drive while stoned. This notion was confirmed by a study of driving capability and cannabinoid ingestion which found that individuals under the influence of cannabinoids tended to refuse to do so when asked whether they would agree to drive.[201]

The paranoia that keeps users from wanting to drive also works to keep those who do decide to drive, careful and attentive. According to the U.S. Department of Transportation, "Under the influence of marijuana, drivers are aware of their impairment, and when the experimental task allows it, they tend to actually decrease speed, avoid passing other cars, and reduce other risk-taking behaviors."[202] As we saw in earlier studies, marijuana users are less likely to have accidents than the general population and the cannabinoid deprivation syndrome seriously impairs balance and movement. Last night's stoner might actually be a better driver today. Despite the fact that marijuana does not profoundly impair driving, it is far better to err on the side of caution and not drive under its influence. There is certainly no question that marijuana can slow reaction time in some users.

But where do we draw the line in the future when more marijuana products are available? What counts as too high to drive? Because it is difficult to assess the levels of cannabinoids in a person's bloodstream without a medical procedure, we will need to develop effective and fair field sobriety tests to measure impairment. And since many people will be using sub-psychoactive therapeutic doses of cannabis products, the current methods of testing urine or saliva for metabolites will not be effective. The only solution is to employ marijuana-specific field sobriety tests. There may well be a market for a device (perhaps similar to a handheld video game) that tests reaction time so that cannabis users can know whether they can safely drive. The best approach, however, is not to drive at all when using marijuana. Plan to wait at least two or three hours after smoking marijuana, or four hours after eating it, before driving. Also (as always) stay off the phone, avoid text messaging, and pay attention to the road and your surroundings whether you've had some marijuana or not. Driving a vehicle is always serious business, and distractions of any sort can lead to tragic consequences.

The question of withdrawal also comes up often in discussions about the relative safety of marijuana. Is there a withdrawal syndrome for marijuana, as there is for opiates? While marijuana is certainly not addictive in the sense that heroin is, chronic, long-term users can experience slight discomfort after suddenly stopping their use. This can include short-term sleep disturbances, restlessness, decreased appetite, mild nausea, or sweating. One interesting thing about these symptoms is that they are remarkably similar to those suffered by the users of rimonabant (the pharmaceutical cannabinoid receptor blocker) before it was pulled from testing and distribution. Is it possible that the abrupt absence of supplemental cannabinoids induces a cannabinoid deprivation syndrome that resembles withdrawal? If all systems of the body regulated by cannabinoids have enough of them and are working in harmony—the appetite is good, sleep is sound, the mood is elevated—is it any surprise that an imbalance results when their levels in the body begin to drop? Perhaps cannabinoid deprivation syndrome is more like malnourishment (as with scurvy or beriberi) than it is like drug withdrawal.

Another lie often told by opponents of legalization is that while not everyone who drinks alcohol does so to get drunk, everyone who smokes marijuana does so to get high. This is sheer nonsense. Alcohol drinkers could just as well have fruit juice if they weren't seeking the psychoactive effects of the alcohol. There are certainly very few people who drink tequila for the taste. What is often forgotten or ignored is that it is just as possible to titrate dosage with marijuana as it is with alcohol. That is, it is perfectly possible to adjust one's marijuana intake in order to get relaxed without being stoned. It may actually be easier to do this with marijuana because it lacks alcohol's tendency to erode users' inhibitions and thereby encourage overconsumption. When marijuana is legal, it will be easier to measure out the proper dosage for what you want because the exact potency will be known.

Treating all marijuana use as abuse serves to generate the type of hysteria necessary for maintaining public support of the War on Drugs. In an effort to generate data that supports its anti-marijuana crusade, NIDA recently appropriated $4 million of taxpayers' money to establish the Center for Cannabis Addiction (CCA), the goal of which is to "develop novel approaches to the prevention, diagnosis, and treatment of marijuana addiction." NIDA will certainly use that $4 million to generate as much nonscientific data as they can—data which will enable the agency to acquire even more funding. After all, while marijuana is not addictive, federal funds are. The DEA, NIDA, and the ONDCP will lie, distort data, and wreck countless lives to keep the money flowing.

NIDA has even invented the deceptive term "cannabis-related disorders" (CRD) in order to justify its parasitic attachment to the federal treasury. A more honest term would be "cannabis deprivation-related disorders" (CDRD). Rather than funding research into cannabinoid therapies, the government is giving NIDA money to "develop safe and effective therapeutic interventions" for marijuana use—all of which, it insists, is abuse. In a boast that betrays NIDA's ignorance about the therapeutic effects of marijuana, officials claim that "recent discoveries about the workings of THC receptors have raised the possibility that scientists may eventually develop a medication that will block THC's intoxicating effects." [203]

The rimonabant debacle clearly shows what can happen when people use cannabinoid receptor blockers: sickness, misery, despair, accidents, and suicide. Spending $4 million developing remedies that do not work for a problem that does not exist is as wasteful as it is irresponsible. Yet NIDA seems to think that it is better to be sick and suicidal than it is to be high. Imagine if this $4 million was instead used by the FDA to find the best way to harness marijuana's natural cannabinoids to prevent and treat Alzheimer's disease? This would be a move away from cruelty and futility, toward justice and health.

> *Do not ask scientists to produce evidence to justify a moral stance. If you don't like what we say about the science then say, 'Okay, we'll take a moral position,' but don't try to tell me the science we've done is wrong!*

If diverting $4 million to the FDA instead of NIDA would be valuable, imagine what could be done with the $4 hundred million budgeted for the ONDCP. With all that money at his disposal, how effective and persuasive has the drug czar been at promulgating his propaganda? After Proposition 215 passed in California, Gen. Barry McCaffrey—a retired general with no medical background—declared war on medical marijuana, saying that there was not a shred of evidence that it was safe and effective. After the public outcry that immediately followed his comments, McCaffrey retreated and appointed a million dollar medical committee to review the matter and confirm his claims. To his disappointment, the committee came back and inferred that the drug czar did not know what he was talking about. How effective has the ONDCP been at suppressing the acceptance of medical marijuana? Since the drug czar first called the movement a "Cheech and Chong show," at least 13 more states have passed medical marijuana laws and 81% of the American people support having access to it.

What could be done with the outrageous $400 million in funds currently allocated to the ONDCP? If we defund the failed Office of National Drug Control Policy and direct research into dangerous drugs and educating the public about their risks to scientists at NIH institutes with a generous $100 million budget, $300 million would be left over for developing effective cannabinoid medicines. Then, consider what diverting even half of the DEA's $2.6 *billion* budget would accomplish. Imagine if $1.3 billion were directed into seeding an entirely new bioscience industry devoted to producing cannabinoid supplements and medicines. NIDA, too, could kick in a chunk of cash from its $1 billion funding request for 2010, and still have plenty of money for researching the truly dangerous substances like tobacco, cocaine, alcohol, opiates and methamphetamine.

So why does the federal government continue to generate pseudoscience and fuel propaganda? The answer is clear: money. The DEA budget has increased from $65 million at its founding in 1972 to $2.6 billion in 2009. Because no administration since the start of the War on Drugs has wanted to appear "soft on drugs," every year the DEA sees its funding increased. In order to keep the money flowing, the DEA, NIDA, and the ONDCP work hard to promote laws and fund programs that increase the number of drug-related arrests, which they in turn use as evidence to justify even more funding.

Arresting marijuana users is an easy way to generate resources for the War on Drugs. Huge amounts of money are directed to local police, who must make enough arrests to justify their annual funding requests. There are also other reasons for local law enforcement's addiction to arresting marijuana users. Sociologist Harry G. Levine of Queen's College conducted an extensive survey of marijuana arrests in New York City and found that local police often have a vested interest in making as many marijuana-related arrests as they can.

Narcotics and patrol police, their supervisors, and others within the NYPD frequently benefit from the marijuana possession arrests. The arrests are relatively safe, easy, and provide training for new officers. The arrests gain overtime pay for patrol and narcotics police and their supervisors. The pot arrests allow officers to show productivity, which counts for promotions and choice assignments. Marijuana arrests enable the NYPD to obtain fingerprints, photographs and other data on young people that they would not otherwise have in their criminal justice databases.[204]

Levine notes that this policy is particularly cruel and unjust because "a marijuana conviction can keep you from getting a student loan, a job, a house or an apartment—even years later." [205]

This carnival of criminal cruelty supports itself by forcibly feeding a portion of the arrestees into drug "treatment" programs. This increases the number of people law enforcement can claim are seeking help for marijuana use. When faced with the choice between jail time and diversion into a treatment program, most people take the easier option. These individuals then become statistics used as evidence that marijuana drives numerous users into drug rehabilitation programs and is therefore dangerous. The truth, however, is that getting assigned to drug treatment for marijuana possession has nothing to do with the user having a marijuana problem—other than having been arrested. Even if you only smoke marijuana once or twice a year and happen to get caught, you can be sent to drug treatment. According to the 2007 *Treatment Episode Data Set Report,* people enrolled in treatment programs for marijuana were twice as likely to have been referred by the criminal justice system as by any other means.

WHO SHOULD NOT USE MARIJUANA

WITH SO MUCH CONVINCING SCIENTIFIC data showing that marijuana is a beneficial substance that supports our health in a number of ways, does this mean that everyone should get stoned? The answer is no: getting high is not appropriate for everyone. But this does not mean that most people could not benefit from using supplemental cannabinoids at a sub-psychoactive level. The anti-carcinogenic and neuroprotective effects of cannabinoids are too valuable to dismiss simply because of THC's psychoactive effects. Expanded access—whether in the form legalization or medicalization—will allow those for whom marijuana's mind-altering qualities are unwanted to obtain strains with fewer psychoactive effects and therefore more value as a medicine.

There is one group of people, however, for whom marijuana in any form may be counterproductive: prospective parents. While there is no convincing evidence that marijuana causes infertility in humans, and no evidence that it affects human reproductive hormones, there is still reason for this group of people to be cautious.[206] One study did find that sperm motility and concentrations were temporarily reduced to the lower range of normal in men who smoked 20 joints per day.[207]

More important, however, is the very slight possibility of early term miscarriage. Normally, the uterus produces huge amounts of the endocannabinoid anandamide for protection, but during the fertility cycle the levels are reduced in order to promote implantation of the fertilized egg. So the reason to avoid marijuana during pregnancy is not because it damages the embryo, but rather because it makes a successful implantation slightly less likely.

How is it that cannabinoids could possibly contribute to early miscarriage? Recall that the components of marijuana inhibit the development, growth, and spread of cancer cells in a variety of ways. One of the ways they stunt tumor growth is by preventing angiogenesis (the production of new blood vessels by cells) by reducing the levels of an angiogenic growth factor, known as VEGF.

During pregnancy, angiogenic growth factors such as VEGF play a strong role in promoting the growth of new blood vessels in the endometrium, decidua, and placenta. It is also recognized that there are striking similarities between tumor growth and the development of the placenta.[208]

In other words, while the reduction in VEGF caused by cannabinoids can help slow the spread of undesirable cells (like cancer); it can also possibly slow the growth of embryonic cells. This is one explanation for how marijuana could theoretically promote spontaneous abortions in early pregnancy. While this effect is not reliable enough for marijuana to be used as a form of birth control, it could possibly frustrate family planning.

It is therefore advisable for prospective parents to avoid using marijuana and cannabis supplements for one or two months before they hope to conceive. It is worth noting, however, that endocannabinoids may also play a positive role in child development. Mothers' milk, for instance, contains large amount of cannabinoids, and blocking CB1 receptors in baby mice causes them to lose their nursing

Prospective Dads, please don't smoke 20 joints per day.

instinct and starve to death. But until we know more about the role of cannabinoids in pregnancy and childbirth, prospective or expecting mothers should avoid using marijuana. That said, pregnant women who have been smoking marijuana have no reason to panic. Despite the theoretical possibility of marijuana inducing an early miscarriage, it is unlikely to do so. One rather small epidemiological study of risk factors in early pregnancy found no definite association between marijuana use and early miscarriage.[209] A 1994 study by the National Toxicology Project also reported that "no adverse genetic effects of THC exposure have been convincingly demonstrated."[210] Still, if you're planning a family, it's better to err on the side of caution and avoid marijuana—along with alcohol, solvents, tobacco, sugar, and fast food.

On the other hand, there may occasionally be a need for some pregnant women to vaporize or smoke small amounts of cannabis to control emesis from severe morning sickness.

Several years ago, a good friend was suffering from unrelenting, torturous, and debilitating morning sickness. The nausea was brutal, and she vomited every time she tried to eat anything. Her inability to eat was causing malnutrition, and the likelihood of a miscarriage was growing every day. In desperation, she turned to marijuana— and after two puffs everything changed. She ate solid food for the first time in weeks. After that, every day or so, she would take one or two puffs and would be able to eat. This was a vital change that saved her pregnancy. I doubt that her daughter, who is now in her twenties and attending graduate school at Columbia University, knows that marijuana saved her life.

As mentioned previously, children, adolescents, and teenagers should not be using marijuana. Science certainly seems to back this up. Although it was questionable in other ways, the previously-mentioned study that inundated adolescent rats with powerful synthetic cannabinoids concluded that "chronic exposure to cannabinoids during adolescence but not during adulthood impairs emotional behavior."[211] Another reason to delay the use of marijuana until adulthood is that its effectiveness against such diseases as head and neck cancer increases significantly with age, especially after age 20.[212]

Above and beyond this, however, there are many behaviors that are reserved for adults because they are just not appropriate for young people—such as gambling, drinking alcohol, sex, unrestricted driving, unsupervised weight training, voting, and so on.

The major reason for restricting children and teenagers from using marijuana, despite its overall positive healthful effects, is simply that it is psychoactive. Although the cognitive and emotional effects of marijuana are useful and often desirable for adults, they present a problem for those who are still growing. Young people have fewer life skills than adults, and are therefore less discreet, more impetuous, and less disciplined. The appeal of marijuana's euphoria can become a consuming distraction for teenagers, rather than a pleasant adjunct to a dynamic life. At a time when young people should be exploring the world and learning the skills they need to live as adults, marijuana use can become a way to avoid dealing with challenges. For them, psychological addiction is a real possibility. Of course, this possibility is not unique to marijuana use. Today, everything from Internet chat to video games to sports can serve as distractions, allowing people to avoid dealing with the demands and challenges of life. It is important to recognize that the young people who seek out marijuana are not necessarily "bad kids." To the contrary, they are often among the most curious and promising youth, seeking respite from the bland and mundane world of institutional education with marijuana's euphoria. When marijuana becomes a problem for these youth, they should not be attacked, vilified, punished, and sent to rehab. They should be taught that becoming an adult is about creating themselves, and that it is their jobs to gather up the raw materials to create wonderful lives for themselves. And if they are doing that while smoking a little weed now and then, it's not a major problem. At least there is no risk of death or brain damage as when young people drink alcohol.

The great American author Norman Mailer once said:

> I always tell my kids—I don't know if they listen or not—that what I think is, get their education first and then start smoking pot. Because what I find is that pot puts things together. Pot is marvelous for getting new connections in the brain. It's divine for that. You think associatively on pot, so you can really have extraordinary thoughts. But the more education you have, the more wonderful connections there are to see in the universe.

When the 20th century's criminalization of cannabis research comes to an end, it might be possible to develop cannabinoid supplements that produce beneficial effects without producing the high. Part of the reason that young people seek out cannabis may be because they are attempting to replenish endocannabinoids that have been depleted by the physical and mental stresses of growing up. If these needs can be met with supplements high in CBD and low in THC, these individuals may actually reduce their marijuana use and reduce the likelihood of abuse. With such promising applications for cannabinoid supplements, it is sad that the development continues to be blocked.

Another group of people who should probably not be getting high are those with life threatening abuse problems. Those struggling with addiction to dangerous drugs should avoid having to contend with yet another mind-altering substance. On the other hand, as previously noted, there are some people who have found that marijuana is a relatively harmless substitute for more dangerous drugs. For them, marijuana could actually help reduce the harms associated with their use of other drugs. An interesting research program would attempt to answer the question of whether low-dose cannabinoid supplements could prevent substance abuse by producing the sense of harmony and well-being that those prone to abuse are seeking. Also, given their neuroprotective and neuroregenerative qualities, it is possible that treatment with cannabinoids could help repair some of the brain damage seen in chronic alcoholics. This is another path of research that deserves attention.

> *If you spend all day doing bong hits and watching reruns of Sponge Bob, then you probably have a marijuana problem.*

Despite its numerous health benefits, there are times when marijuana use can get out of hand. This is the other side of marijuana's benign qualities: Since the euphoria and consciousness alteration that it produces are so pleasant and relatively free of side-effects, there are some who use it too much and too often. Although it does not cause the type of brain damage associated with schizophrenia or psychosis, using too much marijuana can produce what are known as psychotomimetic actions—actions that mimic psychosis. Although Norman Mailer praised marijuana for its enhancement of associative thinking, in exceptionally large quantities those associations can come too quickly and produce delusional notions and beliefs. Of course, this is the case with many drugs, and it is much less likely to happen with marijuana than it is with alcohol, methamphetamine, cocaine, or heroin.

A friend gave me permission to relate the story of his brother's experience with marijuana abuse. "Dr. Jim" (as I will call him) is a dentist who had to give up marijuana because his use had gotten out of hand and was beginning to threaten his career. Dr. Jim would smoke a joint while driving to work in the morning, followed by several more throughout the day between appointments. While his marijuana use was not seriously impacting the quality of his work, the strange and disjointed conversations he would initiate with his patients were beginning to raise eyebrows. It seemed that his already nervous patients did not appreciate the stream-of-consciousness monologues that Dr. Jim would launch into while he worked, and it was beginning to hurt his practice. Questions were asked, and eventually a patient threatened to report him to the state dental board. Dr. Jim's family decided to hold an intervention, he stopped using marijuana, and he joined a support group for medical professionals with a marijuana problem. Once again the question arises: Could sub-psychoactive cannabinoid supplements help keep Dr. Jim from returning to marijuana abuse?

Not everyone who uses marijuana chronically has a problem with it. Irv Rosenfeld, one of the few remaining participants in the Compassionate IND program, smokes about a dozen joints every day and is a successful stockbroker who teaches sailing to the physically challenged. Even Louis Armstrong, the architect of American jazz, smoked five cigar-sized joints every day. Some people may experience more severe forms of endocannabinoid deficiency and be able to ingest constantly without losing motivation, skills or vitality.

In order to assess whether you have a problem with marijuana, it is useful to occasionally conduct a personal inventory. This means asking yourself a series of questions about how using marijuana fits into your life, such as:

- Are you happy with your life? Are you keeping fit, eating nourishing food, and staying away from high sugar, high fat junk food?
- Are you pulling your weight? If you are in school, are you getting acceptable grades? Are you a reliable employee? Are you helping to make a better home for your family?
- Are you taking care of necessities? Is the dog walked? Are the bills paid? And what about the dishes in the sink?
- Are you learning new skills and information? Do you have a broad range of interests and pursuits? Is marijuana fueling your curiosity and passion for living?

- Do you have loving interpersonal relationships with family and a trusted group of friends?
- Do you do something that takes you outside of your self-absorption? Have you worked for a cause you believe in or volunteered to help others?

Notice that only a few elements in this personal inventory address marijuana directly. This type of self-review is a good idea for people who are prone to overindulgence, whether in Internet trolling, video games, religion, television, or sports. Just remember, if you spend all day doing bong hits and watching reruns of SpongeBob, then you probably have a marijuana problem.

Problems arise when so-called experts define any level of marijuana use as abuse. It is perfectly possible to smoke marijuana every day, as many people do, and not have a problem with it. This has been our cultural experience with alcohol. My father, for example, enjoyed one or two cocktails every night after work before dinner and never had a problem with alcohol. He was a great provider and family man who was involved in numerous civic projects and remains physically and mentally active even in his mid-80s. If alcohol, which is a more harmful and addictive, less beneficial substance, can be used responsibly, why should using marijuana automatically be labeled as abuse?

The Marijuana Renaissance

IT IS A REMARKABLE TIME for both the biological and the social sciences. In a very real way, scientific research on cannabis and cannabinoids is expanding and rewriting our knowledge of how our bodies function and how to keep them in a state of optimum health. An enormous body of scientific data now reveals that using marijuana is good for us—apparently very good for us. This new perspective will certainly generate an enormous increase in marijuana's popularity as the scientific data about its benefits continues to overshadow the myths about its dangers. So the questions arise: How do we move from a culture of cannabis prohibition to one that acknowledges and facilitates its responsible use? Will drug warriors and their allies cling to their delusions in a desperate attempt to preserve prohibition, or will they admit failure and redirect their efforts to help relieve suffering and optimize health by allowing marijuana to be used appropriately?

Following the passage of the first medical marijuana ballot proposition in California in 1996, various models of commercial cannabis production, development, and distribution emerged. Since Dennis Peron founded the first buyers' club in a small studio apartment, dispensaries have proliferated throughout California and Colorado. When Colorado began accepting applications for medical marijuana vendors, the officials in charge were avalanched with an average of 500 submissions arriving daily. The number of commercial cannabis outlets jumped from 12 to 1000, and currently there are more marijuana shops in Denver than there are liquor stores and Starbucks combined.

The incredible success of commercial marijuana dispensaries in areas where they are tolerated or embraced speaks to the enormous and previously underestimated popularity of marijuana. People enjoy using marijuana because of its ability to produce a profound sense of mental and physical well-being. As we saw in preceding chapters, this sensation is not a harmful intoxication, such as alcohol causes, but rather a healthy biochemical response to the activity of supplemental cannabinoids. It is therefore understandable that human beings have revered the cannabis plant throughout history.

Wherever marijuana is permitted to move from the criminal underground into mainstream commerce, its enormous appeal becomes apparent. A celebrity substance abuse consultant said that it is "interesting that when I treat people for multiple substances—cocaine, alcohol, and pot—the one they really miss is the pot... The euphoria from the drug creates sort of a love-type reaction—they love the drug—it's a nurturing, sort of warm feeling they can't get any other way." The doctor is right. Marijuana is the only effective source for the compounds that activate our cannabinoid receptors, improve our health, and thereby give us a greater sense of happiness and calm.

An impressive example of a professionally-run cannabis dispensary is Harborside Health Center in Oakland, California. This pioneering business was prominently featured in a *Fortune* magazine cover story entitled "Is Pot Already Legal?" and according to founder Steve DeAngelo it serves as an example of how to "flip the switch" from prohibition to legality. The ways and means of production and distribution are already in place, and all that remains to make it legal for adults is to remove the requirement of a doctor's recommendation.

Marijuana commerce is becoming respectable. Harborside is featured on the Oakland Chamber of Commerce's web site as a legitimate and valued member of the city's business community. When the company opened an additional center in San Jose, members of the city's Chamber of Commerce attended the ribbon cutting.

Harborside has joined together the community center and pharmacy models of medical marijuana distribution in a bright, clean, and inviting facility. After passing through security upon entering the building, patients proceed into a large room where they line up for service in front of counters which at first glance look like a bank branch or a car rental facility. A closer look reveals that each counter has a glass case displaying a number of neatly-arranged varieties of marijuana, all labeled according to their potency, as well as several types of hashish and edible goods. The sales counters are staffed by "budtenders" who are trained to understand the appropriate applications for various strains of cannabis. Patients even earn a free gram when they fill up their frequent buyer's punch card. Stacked neatly on the other side of the room are racks and racks of starter plants of several varieties for sale to those who wish to grow their own. Harborside also has meeting and treatment rooms where members can avail themselves of support groups, healthy-living classes, and bodywork therapy. The staff encourages and facilitates activism by rewarding members with a gram of buds for every half hour of pro-marijuana lobbying and letter writing.

One of the best things about legitimizing the marijuana business is that it allows for the development of quality-control standards. At Harborside and a growing number of other dispensaries, display samples are presented in bright, well-lit cases and labeled with the amount of THC and CBD they each contain. In order to determine the potency and purity of the marijuana, dispensaries are sending samples out for testing at facilities like Steep Hill Lab. Similar testing labs are arising to provide analytical services to medical marijuana providers in other parts of California as well as in Colorado. Unfortunately, the Colorado testing facility Full Spectrum Laboratories in Denver was raided by the DEA and shut down.

Overall, the leniency of the laws in California and Colorado has allowed an entirely new industry to arise from the immense demand for medical marijuana. With California mired in debt and stagnation, the marijuana industry seems to be the only one that is flourishing in the state. Analytical facilities like Steep Hill Lab have become vital to the legitimacy of this growing industry. The directors of the lab were kind enough to allow me to submit some samples of marijuana for potency testing so that I could see how their process works. I brought two samples that a friend had grown for patients in northern California: one was a mild strain known as "Halo" and the other was a more potent one with the unfortunate name "DOA." A more appropriate name might be "VOA," vital on arrival.

Each sample was macerated by hand with clean stainless steel scissors before being placed into a vial containing a solvent solution. The vial was then placed into a "sonicator," which sends sound waves through the solution which vibrate the cell membranes until they rupture, speeding up the analysis. A portion of the solution was then placed into the gas chromatography unit. At this point, the process became extremely technical, but seemed to proceed as follows: The solution was vaporized and sent through a flame ionization unit, which measures how well the sample conducts electricity by passing it through a hydrogen flame and charts the results. The peaks of the chart reveal the ratio of the cannabinoids THC, CBD, and CBN in the sample. The Halo strain registered 7.78 percent THC with only 0.23 percent CBD and

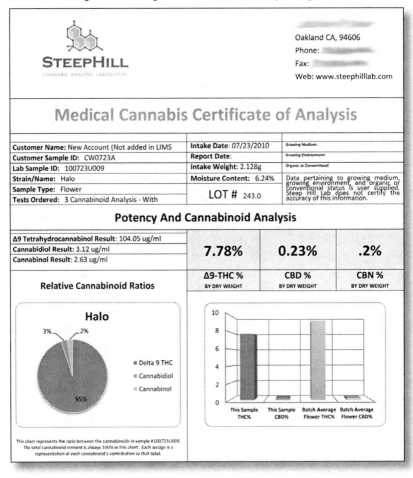

STEEPHILL
CANNABIS ANALYSIS LABORATORY

Oakland CA, 94606
Phone:
Fax:
Web: www.steephilllab.com

Medical Cannabis Certificate of Analysis

Customer Name: New Account (Not added in LIMS	**Intake Date:** 07/23/2010	Growing Medium:
Customer Sample ID: CW0723A	**Report Date:**	Growing Environment:
Lab Sample ID: 100723U009	**Intake Weight:** 2.128g	Organic or Conventional
Strain/Name: Halo	**Moisture Content:** 6.24%	Data pertaining to growing medium, growing environment, and organic or conventional status is user supplied. Steep Hill Lab does not certify the accuracy of this information.
Sample Type: Flower	**LOT #** 243.0	
Tests Ordered: 3 Cannabinoid Analysis - With		

Potency And Cannabinoid Analysis

Δ9 Tetrahydrocannabinol Result: 104.05 ug/ml Cannabidiol Result: 3.12 ug/ml Cannabinol Result: 2.63 ug/ml	**7.78%**	**0.23%**	**.2%**
Relative Cannabinoid Ratios	Δ9-THC % BY DRY WEIGHT	CBD % BY DRY WEIGHT	CBN % BY DRY WEIGHT

Halo
3%   2%
95%
■ Delta 9 THC
■ Cannabidiol
■ Cannabinol

This chart represents the ratio between the cannabinoids in sample #100723U009. The total cannabinoid content is always 100% in this chart. Each wedge is a representation of each cannabinoid's contribution to that total.

This Sample THC% — This Sample CBD% — Batch Average Flower THC% — Batch Average Flower CBD%

0.20 percent CBN (see chart). The DOA strain registered 10.79 percent THC with 0.24 and 0.19 percents CBD and CBN respectively.

When more detailed analyses are requested (for anything from terpenoid levels to pesticide residue) the vaporized sample material is also sent through a mass spectrometer, which analyzes the mass of the particles and separates them into a spectrum using quartz covered in gold—it really sounds like alchemy and would probably require a weekend tutorial to fully comprehend. Yet the lab is able to process about 100 samples per day, though sometimes it takes longer (such as when samples must be incubated when testing for pathogens such as harmful mold).

Despite the claims of drug warriors, not everyone who uses marijuana does so to get stoned. Some just want to relax, reduce their pain, or just get a case of the giggles or munchies. There is a continuum running from relaxed to high to stoned. Knowing that a strain of marijuana has 7.78 percent THC is better for those who prefer not to be high or stoned than one with 10.79 percent THC. It is now possible to buy strains of cannabis at certain dispensaries that have more CBD than THC, which provide various kinds of relief and protection with few or no mind-altering effects. Having this knowledge eliminates the need to do a lot of hit-or-miss experimentation and allows users to quickly select the types of cannabis products most appropriate for their health care needs.

Complementing the dispensaries and the labs are medical marijuana delivery services, which cater to those who are unable or unwilling to visit a storefront. The convenience is certainly hard to beat: The patient goes online or makes a phone call and selects from a menu of items which are then brought to their front door. The patient shows the appropriate certification, pays, and receives the order. In San Francisco, the Green Cross delivery service offers over a dozen popular strains of lab-analyzed marijuana as well as everything from mint THC tincture spray and THC-infused body balm to THC gel caps and a wide assortment of edibles. Orders placed early in the day frequently include a free edible and the delivery is usually made in less than an hour.

The emergence of this medical marijuana industry has created a demand for a diverse cannabis service sector which includes breeders, growers, graders, testers, consultants, merchandisers, vendors, and an enormous support staff of bud trimmers, transporters, budtenders, bakers, and so on. In 2007, Richard Lee founded Oaksterdam University in an economically-depressed area of Oakland, California, in order to help meet the demand for these workers and establish something of a professional standard.

Lee ran a city-approved dispensary for several years before deciding to start an industry training program. The original "campus" was in a long-vacant storefront, but Oaksterdam now offers its "Quality Training for the Cannabis Industry" in a 30,000-square-foot building in the same area. Classes include Dispensary Operations, Patient Relations, Procurement and Allotment, Federal vs. State Law, Legal Rights, the Science of Cannabis, Horticulture 101, Methods of Ingesting, and History and Politics. As of September 2010, over 12,000 students have trained at Oaksterdam, and there are also additional campuses in Los Angeles, Michigan, and elsewhere in Northern California.

Lee's constellation of "cannabusinesses" has revitalized the down-trodden area of Oakland and provided him with the financial resources to launch Proposition 19, a state ballot initiative that sought to legalize marijuana for adult recreational use in California in 2010. The campaign for Proposition 19 brought an enormous amount of media attention to the issue of legalizing and taxing marijuana. Although it lost by 7 percentage points, the measure ignited a serious discussion about the issue. And even though it failed to pass, over 4.5 million voters in California said "yes" to the legalization of marijuana. That's more votes than Meg Whitman got for the $160 million dollars she spent in her run for governor of California, as well as more votes than either candidate for Attorney General received.

In July 2010, the Oakland City Council approved a 45,000 square foot indoor marijuana growing facility that could produce up to 70,000 pounds of cannabis (grown in artificial light and fed by a solution of chemical nutrients) per year. Still, even if California does legalize marijuana, federal laws against marijuana cultivation would remain the same, and the proprietor would be in danger of spending a long time in federal custody. In fact a warning letter from the DEA prompted the city to rescind its approval for the business in early 2011.

In 1999, I was fortunate enough to be given a tour of an enormous legal cannabis cultivation operation. In acres and acres of greenhouses in the English countryside, British company GW Pharmaceuticals grows an enormous volume of marijuana for use in manufacturing their cannabinoid-based drug Sativex. The first thing I noticed as I approached the entrance was a faint but detectable and enticingly familiar "skunky" scent. The building complex is immense and is comprised of a series of warehouse-sized greenhouses. The plants are cultivated on waist-high tables and are rooted in a special material that looks likes shredded Spanish moss. They are fed with a nutrient solution and grown with a combination of natural and artificial light—a necessity given the frequently overcast skies in the area. The plants are grown from cuttings taken from large "mothers" and are cultivated using a method known as "sea of green." The cuttings are rooted and grown under nearly continuous light until they are about a foot tall, at which point they are subjected to light deprivation. This change triggers the budding cycle and speeds up the maturation of the flowers. When it is time to initiate budding, giant metallic screens are unfolded, shrouding the farm in darkness. The strange sight and clacking sound of acres of screens unfolding uniformly over an ocean of cannabis plants is a most impressive experience.

GW Pharmaceuticals cultivates a variety of strains with different cannabinoid profiles. The company is on the cutting edge of cannabinoid medicine development and is researching different cannabinoid mixtures to find which work most efficiently for which ailments. The company extracts the cannabinoids from the plant material and stores the concentrate in liquid nitrogen until needed. The final product is an alcohol-based spray that is administered under the tongue where the cannabinoids are absorbed into the bloodstream. This works faster than eating marijuana, but slower than inhaling it. The THC is blended with CBD, tempering the spray's psychoactive effects and allowing some patients to titrate their dosage in a way that produces relief without inducing a high. The delivery system can also be programmed by prescribing physicians to yield a specific number of doses within a limited time frame, which is believed to reduce the black market demand for the drug.

One possible concern about Sativex is its use of alcohol as a delivery medium. Due to alcohol's carcinogenic effects on oral tissue, could frequent and long-term Sativex users be exposed to an increased risk of cancer? Ethan Russo dismisses the risk as less than that for daily users of mouthwash. Someone with a long-term need for cannabinoids at a sub-psychoactive level who is bothered by alcohol might consider vaporizing a lower-potency strain. Because some patients have an aversion to alcohol some dispensaries have begun selling tinctures made with glycerin.

✳

Many smaller cannabis cultivators fear legalization out of concern that they would be unable to survive once large-scale producers are established. With de facto legalization in California by way of medical marijuana, prices have dropped significantly, and some cultivators worry that their profits will continue to decline. Yet others feel that the more adept cultivators will still have a customer base. There may well be a large market for exotic and exceptional marijuana strains, just as there are large numbers of consumers willing to pay more for organic, farmer's market quality produce despite the widespread availability of cheaper fruits and vegetables.

Opponents of legalization protest that the tax revenue from legalized marijuana will be insignificant because anyone will be permitted to grow it. This is a misconception. Although cannabis is a tenacious, weed-like plant; it does not produce market-grade marijuana without a lot of attention and dedication. In addition, there are a number of things that can go wrong and ruin a crop. Yet consumers will want top-grade products and will appreciate the convenience of buying an ounce of above-average or connoisseur-grade marijuana. Smaller boutique growers will therefore still find a market. The best will thrive.

After legalization fewer growers will be forced to grow cannabis indoors. When the laws against marijuana use, distribution, and production are repealed, cannabis will be able to come out of the closet—literally. The cultivation of cannabis will emerge from hidden basements, closets, attics, and secret rooms filled with high intensity lights and liquefied nutrients washing over soilless roots. Growing indoors is a resource-draining pursuit necessitated by prohibition and sometimes environment.

It is impossible to replicate the unique qualities of sunlight in a basement. While it is possible to artificially manipulate the light in order to alter the plant's growth cycle and shock it into rapidly producing generous amounts of resin, the holistic qualities of these plants are ultimately inferior to those of well-grown outdoor cannabis. Project CBD, for example, found significantly higher levels of CBD in cannabis grown outdoors. Also, we can logically extrapolate from a study of strawberries that organic marijuana, grown in natural light will have a greater concentration of healing compounds. That study, conducted by scientists at Washington State University determined that, "organic strawberries had significantly higher antioxidant activity and concentrations of ascorbic acid and phenolic compounds." [213]

There is justified speculation that the flavonoids in cannabis help to temper some of the side-effects of THC, thus making the experience of smoking marijuana more pleasurable and healing. These compounds are evidently greater in cannabis grown outdoors. When the price of marijuana drops after legalization, growing indoors may become a less viable business model due to the cost of the energy and equipment it requires. But indoor cultivation will remain the only option for cannabis lovers in areas with adverse weather conditions such as Colorado and the Netherlands.

The natural flowering of the cannabis plant unfolds over several months as the days shorten. Outdoor plants—bathed in natural sunlight, roots buried in soil, caressed by the breeze—ease their way into the flowering phase, increasing this activity in harmony with the cycles of the sun, earth, and moon. Indoor plants are by contrast shocked into the flowering phase as they are abruptly reduced from 18 hours or more to just 12 hours of artificial light. Though many indoor crops have wonderful qualities, even the best lack the superlative traits found in outdoor cannabis. Unfortunately, some hydroponically-grown indoor marijuana reflects this unnatural growing environment in its effects, producing a sudden and stupefying high that can leave novice users feeling ill and paranoid. This tends to give opponents of legalization a false foundation for their claims about the "new marijuana." Of course, indoor marijuana is not new; it is just extremely psychoactive and may lack some healthful compounds that harmonize the high. Interestingly, legalization may be the best way to reduce or eliminate such cannabis by reducing indoor growing.

The legal cultivation of cannabis will probably follow several models. There will be mass production facilities—both outdoor farms and greenhouses like GW Pharmaceuticals' facility—growing commercial-grade cannabis. There will also be smaller farms that specialize in growing varieties that require more attention and skill. And there will be farms that specialize in signature or branded strains that they have developed themselves. The most distinctive of these will find loyal customers in the same way that microbrews thrive alongside large-scale corporate beer brands.

Once the law catches up with the science of marijuana, a huge variety of healthful products will be made available. At some of the medical dispensaries in California the selection of cannabis products is already stunning and amusing. There is everything from peanut butter to salad dressing and soda pop as well as "pot tart" pastries and commercial candy knockoffs like "reefers peanut butter cup"—all of which have been infused with cannabinoids.

With the threat of incarceration removed, effective research and development will accelerate and new supplements will be formulated to address specific health-care needs. Someone with a family history of Alzheimer's, cancer, or other illnesses could perhaps stop into a dispensary and purchase their supply of high-CBD marijuana. An encapsulated blend of CBD, THC, and vitamin D_3 might be employed by those at risk of MS. Patients showing early symptoms of diabetes, Alzheimer's, or other illnesses could be placed on cannabinoid supplements from plants hybridized to generate appropriate levels of terpenoids and flavonoids for keeping such syndromes suppressed.

Post-legalization, we will likely see cannabis bars and vapor lounges arise and begin to compete with liquor bars as gathering places for relaxation and levity. This displacement of alcohol will save millions in public dollars now used for treating the diseases and injuries associated with drinking. As we have seen, encouraging the consumption of marijuana at the remaining bars will also help to prevent brain damage from alcohol toxicity.

Sales of psychoactive cannabis products would be limited to adults, with the exception of minors with a physician's recommendation or prescription. Since it is permissible in 23 states for parents to provide alcohol to their underage children, the same policy should apply to marijuana. Certainly no one in their right mind would condone getting a child drunk or high, but some responsible parents do allow their children to partake of small amounts of alcohol or marijuana on special occasions or for special religious or social rituals.

Vaporization will grow in popularity as more affordable, efficient, and portable devices are engineered. With the proliferation of vaporization, smoking marijuana will become less evident in public areas. The laws against the smoking of tobacco will likely apply to marijuana even though combusted cannabis is far less harmful than cigarette smoke. No one should be put at risk of becoming unwillingly high, but there should be less stringent restrictions on where one can vaporize since it does not produce any second-hand smoke.

When it comes to traffic laws, effective field sobriety tests specific to marijuana can and should be developed, as the unique nature of cannabinoids makes lab testing a pointless task. Since the cannabinoid metabolites that urine or saliva tests currently measure can persist for up to 30 days in regular users, these methods will not work to detect impairment at the time of arrest. When large numbers of people are using cannabinoid products for health (frequently without getting high), these tests will have to be discarded and replaced with field sobriety tests appropriate for drivers who appear impaired.

What the drug warriors feared most about legal medical marijuana has come to pass: many thousands of people have come out of the closet as cannabis users, normalizing the activity in the eyes of much of the general public. The scorn and derision that Nancy Reagan and her cohorts worked so hard to attach to marijuana use is quickly becoming a relic of an ignorant and bygone era. The world's greatest Olympian athlete was recently photographed taking a bong hit, and the public turned not on him but on the cereal manufacturer that dropped him as spokesperson. A World Series winning Major League pitcher was pulled over while driving and found to have a pipe and some buds, and no one was outraged. Instead, T-shirts began appearing with "Let Tim Smoke" printed over a marijuana leaf. Rapper and hip-hop mogul Snoop Dogg joined Martha Stewart on her show to bake some "green brownies," allowing Snoop Dogg to complain that they did not have the most important ingredient. Martha laughed, the audience laughed, and we continue to walk away from prohibition.

Attitudes are changing quickly. Fashion magazine *Marie Claire* published a story on "Stiletto Stoners," over-achieving professional women who like to cut their stress levels with a few puffs of marijuana instead of the traditional cocktail. *The TODAY Show* ran an interview with the editor, Joanne Coles and psychiatrist Dr. Julie Holland for the obligatory opposing view. When interviewer Matt Lauer turned to Dr. Holland for the "darker side of this issue" Holland replied:

> It's very different from alcohol. It's more of a mind drug. I feel alcohol is more of a deadening, numbing, more like a body drug. People are unwinding and they are relaxing but they're also able to think and maybe analyze or think more clearly—maybe pull back and see the macro, maybe make some changes. I think cannabis is more of a psychotherapeutic drug than alcohol is, it could be more helpful in their lives... I think the behavior should be normalized.[214]

As public awareness grows about cannabis' health-protective qualities, social disapproval for marijuana use will continue to fade.

Attitudes regarding marijuana use are beginning to conform to reality. The celebration of marijuana culture on April 20 or 420 has become an unofficial party holiday, a sort of stoner's St. Patrick's Day. The numerous smoke-in gatherings that occur across the country are framed by the national media not as a social problem but as a quirky aspect of our American culture.

During the height of the Drug War under Reagan and the first Bush, marijuana was strategically demonized through connection with the new and devastating crack cocaine crisis. The association was intended to promulgate a "zero tolerance" attitude toward all mind-altering substances other than caffeine, alcohol, and nicotine. Any realistic or lighthearted reference to using marijuana was prohibited—not by law but by governmental pressure and propaganda.

Federal agencies pushed and bribed television and film producers to incorporate storylines about the horrors of marijuana use into their programming because the culture was to be scrubbed clean of any amusing reference to marijuana. In an episode of 1970s police sitcom *Barney Miller*, an older detective accidentally eats a hash brownie seized as evidence in a bust. "The first time in twenty years that I feel really great and it has to be illegal," he remarks. When another officer is told to get the brownies tested for pot, he starts to eat one and is reprimanded "Not that way!" During the Reagan years, the episode was pulled from syndication and banned from being broadcast lest it send a bad message to the youth. Similarly, the 1980 film *Cheech and Chong's*

Next Movie was edited so that a bag of Thai sticks became a bag of diamonds and every possible marijuana or drug reference was excised.

Even the comedic portrayal of marijuana users has changed. The heirs to Cheech and Chong's stoner shtick are not frumpy, dull-witted clowns but rather Harold and Kumar, a young business executive and a reluctant medical school student. And Cheech and Chong have reunited in the wake of Harold and Kumar's successful films. Robin Williams comforted Conan O'Brian over his loss of *The Tonight Show* by telling him to "take a good long toke." On-air radio personalities admit smoking a joint before watching *Avatar* and fewer and fewer people consider adults getting high to be a social problem or concern.

After signing a bill that would reduce the penalty for the recreational use of marijuana from a misdemeanor to a civil infraction in California, Governor Arnold Schwarzenegger told Jay Leno that, "no one cares if you smoke a joint or not." In conservative Montana, prospective jurors staged a "mutiny," that led the judge in a marijuana possession case to admit, "Geeze, I don't know if we can seat a jury." A plea agreement was reached after the prosecutor concluded that public opinion "is not supportive of the state's marijuana law and appeared to prevent any conviction from being obtained."

Iowa's 7th District Senior Associate Judge Douglass MacDonald spoke out for legalization and said that marijuana is "no big deal" because "it doesn't cause people to do bad things."

Smoking marijuana is no longer considered to be bad behavior. There are, however, those who have not received the message and who continue to marinate in marijuanaphobia and euphoranoia. The 2009 film *It's Complicated* received an "R" rating (restricting admission to adults or minors with a guardian) solely because it features a scene with Steve Martin and Meryl Streep enjoying a joint "without any negative consequences." If they had been arrested or gunned down by drug lords, the film could have been given a "PG-13" rating. If someone makes a documentary of this book, would it be rated "R" because it promotes marijuana use to protect us from serious illnesses?

The baby boomers—the first sizable American demographic to use large amounts of marijuana—are rediscovering that using marijuana is fun and also helpful for relieving many of the aches and pains that come with ageing. Researchers from Ohio State found that marijuana "may offer [memory] protection by reducing inflammation and by restoring neurogenesis."[215] They also concluded that "later in life marijuana might actually help your brain" and that "it takes very little marijuana to produce benefits in the older brain."[216] Dr. Yannick Marchalant says that for older individuals "a puff is enough" because "a single puff each day is necessary to produce significant benefit."[217]

But the prohibitionists will not leave you alone. If you thought you were done with urine testing after retirement, think again. A survey by the U.S. Substance Abuse and Mental Health Services Administration (SAMHSA) found that 8.5 percent of men between the ages of 50 and 54 have used marijuana in the past year.[218] The agency erroneously labels this increase in marijuana use as "substance abuse," with SAMHSA Administrator Pamela S. Hyde proclaiming that there is a need to "establish improved screening and appropriate referral to treatment as part of routine health care services."[219] Hyde apparently believes that holding individuals' access to health care

> *A puff is enough because a single puff each day is necessary to produce significant benefit."*

hostage will force them to abstain from using marijuana—regardless of the fact that ingesting it actually decreases the likelihood of developing a number of serious and costly illnesses. Once the older generation learns that using marijuana reduces their odds of getting a huge range of serious illnesses, the number of cannabis consumers will really grow—and that's a good thing.

Despite the worst efforts of the straggling remnants of the reefer madness crowd, the marijuana renaissance is entering full bloom. This change in attitude and direction is fully supported by a solid and growing body of scientific evidence. Curiosity about how marijuana works has led to some truly revolutionary discoveries about the nature and function of many of our biological systems. Investigating the endocannabinoid system has revealed that the products of the cannabis plant really do have the amazing healing properties ascribed to it for thousands of years.

Although we are only in the early stages of the cannabinoids and health revolution, as our body of knowledge expands we are gaining a broader understanding of the properties of the many therapeutic compounds in marijuana and how they interact. Cannabis is already being cultivated for specific therapeutic purposes in states that allow medical use, and this is only going to get better.

It is time to redefine our society's relationship with marijuana as a scientific one. We should return to the days before the Marihuana Tax Act when cannabis remedies were available and marijuana was not criminalized. The health advantages conferred upon its users by marijuana are now undeniably supported by science, and it is high time that public policy reflects reality. Using the threat of arrest and imprisonment to deprive people of a substance that brings joy and protects them against disease is cruel and unusual behavior. The new science surrounding marijuana and cannabinoids is so profound that even some of the most ardent of the prohibitionist organizations are beginning to admit what the research is revealing. As noted in Chapter 18, NIDA has consistently claimed that marijuana "increases the risk of cancer of the head, neck and lung" as well as "emphysema."[220] Upon revisiting that website, it was almost shocking to see that NIDA has dropped those false claims and replaced them with text stating that "a recent case-controlled study found no positive associations between marijuana use and lung, upper respiratory or upper digestive tract cancers. Thus, the link between marijuana smoking and these cancers remains unsubstantiated at this time."[221] Despite this revision, the agency is not quite ready to publicly admit that marijuana protects us from these diseases.

Should you use marijuana? If you're an adult, and you want to be healthier, the answer is probably yes. If you have a history of Alzheimer's disease or cancer in your family, using cannabinoid products might be a good idea. You don't even need to smoke it: you could vaporize it or eat it. You don't need to use a lot, and you don't have to get stoned but you should probably use a small amount every day, because as the French researcher Dr. Yannick Marchalant says "a puff is enough." Remember that one toke a day is good advice according to Alzheimer's researcher Gary Wenk "because it appears as though only a single puff each day is necessary to produce significant benefit."[222]

Getting high or stoned is not a problem as long as it is done responsibly. You won't hurt your liver and you won't die of an overdose, but you will protect yourself from cancer and dementia. Recall that the

NTP study found that the more THC that rats and mice ingested, the longer they lived.

So, ask the drug warriors and prohibitionists: Marijuana discourages the development and progression of lung cancer, head and neck cancers, colon cancer, pancreatic cancer, other cancers, Alzheimer's disease, ALS, Parkinson's disease, and brain damage from alcohol. It creates healthy new brain cells, it protects us from injury, it makes sex more enjoyable, it makes eating more pleasurable, it makes going to a museum a revelation, so why shouldn't we be using it?

END NOTES

Chapter 1

1   Mechoulam, R., "The Cannabinoid System in Neuroprotection," lecture, Third National Clinical Conference on Cannabis Therapeutics, Charlottesville, VA, (May 20-22, 2004).

2   "Conversation with Raphael Mechoulam," *Addiction* 102: 6 (June, 2007): 887-893.

3   Ibid.

4   Ibid.

5   Mechoulam, R., "The Cannabinoid System in Neuroprotection".

6   Iverson, Leslie, "Forward," in *Cannabis and Cannabinoids: Pharmacology, Toxicology and Therapeutic Potential*, edited by Franjo Grotenhermen, M.D., and Ethan Russo, M.D. (Binghamton, NY: The Haworth Integrated Healing Press, 2002): xxii.

7   Pollan, Michael, *The Botany of Desire* (New York: Random House, 2001): 154.

8   Brady, Pete, "Dr. Ethan Russo: Pot Pioneer". www.maps.org/media/potpioneer.html (accessed February, 2011)

Chapter 2

9   Munson, A.E., et al., "Anticancer Activity of Cannabinoids," *Journal of the National Cancer Institute* 55 (September, 1975): 597.

10   Ibid.

11   U.S. Department of Health and Human Services, Public Health Service, National Institutes of Health, *NTP Technical Report on the Toxicology*

and Carcinogenesis Studies of 1-Trans-Delta9-Tetrahydrocannabinol in F344/N Rats and B6C3F1 Mice (Gavage Studies) (Washington, D.C.: 1994): 7.

12   Swerdlow, Lanny, "Interview With Donald Tashkin, M.D.," Marijuana Compassion and Common Sense, show # 024 season 1. www.youtube.com/watch?v=LMFi3VQbDhg (accessed February, 2011).

13   Hashibe, Mia et al., "Marijuana Use and the Risk of Lung and Upper Aerodigestive Tract Cancers: Results of a Population-Based Case-Control Study," *Cancer Epidemiological, Biomarkers and Prevention* 5 (October, 2006): 1829-1834.

14   Snerdlow, L.

15   Zimm, Angela, "Marijuana Stops Growth of Lung Cancer Tumors in Mice," *Bloomberg News* (April 17, 2007). [URL] boards.cannabis.com/current-events/112410-marijuana-stops-growth-lung-cancer-tumors-mice.html (accessed February, 2011).

16   Hashibe, Mia, et al.

17   McManis, Sam, "Legalize It? Medical Evidence on Marijuana Blows Both Ways," *The Sacramento Bee*, (March 12, 2010): 1.

Chapter 3

18   Nuland, Sherwin, *How We Die* (New York: Alfred A. Knopf, 1994): 207.

19   Abrams, Donald and Guzman, Manuel, "Cannabis and Cancer" in *Integrative Oncology*, edited by Donald Abrams and Andrew Weil (New York: Oxford University Press, 2009).

20   Ibid.

21   Chianchi, Fabio, et al., "Cannabinoid receptor activation induces apoptosis through tumor necrosis factor alpha-mediated ceramide de novo synthesis in colon cancer cells," *Clinical Cancer Research* 14 (December 1, 2008): 7691-7700. www.ncbi.nlm.nih.gov/pubmed/19047095 (accessed February, 2011).

22   Medveczky, Maria M., et al., "Delta-9-THC inhibits lytic replication of gamma oncogenic herpesviruses in vitro," *BMC Medicine* 2 (2004).

23   Ramer, Robert, Burkhard Hinz, "Inhibition of Cancer Cell Invasion by Cannabinoids via Increased Expression of Tissue Inhibitor of Matrix Metalloproteinases-1," *Journal of National Cancer Institute* 100: 1 (December 25, 2007): 59-69.

24 Gustafsson, K., et al., "Expression of cannabinoid receptors type 1 and type 2 in non-Hodgkin lymphoma: growth inhibition by receptor activation," *International Journal of Cancer* 123 (September 1, 2008): 1025-33.

25 Holly, Elizabeth A., et al., "Case-Controlled Study of Non-Hodgkin's Lymphoma Among Women and Heterosexual Men in the San Francisco Bay Area, California," *American Journal of Epidemiology* 150 (August 15, 1999): 375-89.

26 Christina Blazquez, et al. "Inhibition of tumor angiogenesis by cannabinoids," *The FASEB Journal* 17 (January 2, 2003): 529-531.

27 Llanos Casanova, M., et al., "Inhibition of skin tumor growth and angiogenesis in vivo by activation of cannabinoid receptors," *Journal of Clinical Investigation* 111 (January 1, 2003): 43-50.

28 Guzman, Manuel, personal correspondence, January 18, 2010.

29 Guzman, Manuel, "Cannabinoids: Potential Anticancer Agents," *Nature Reviews* 3 (October 2003): 751.

30 Olea-Herrero, N., et al., "Inhibition of human tumour prostate PC-3 cell growth by cannabinoids R(+)-Methanandamide and JWH-015: Involvement of CB2," *British Journal of Cancer* 101, (2009): 940-950.

31 Ruiz, Lidia, et al. "Delta-9-THC induces apoptosis in human prostate PC-3 cells via a receptor-independent mechanism," FEBS *Letters* 458 (September 24, 1999): 400-404. (Federation of European Biochemical Societies)

32 Leelawat, s. et al., "The dual effects of delta(9)-tetrahydrocannabinol on cholangiocarcinoma cells: anti-invasion activity at low concentration and apoptosis induction at high concentration." *Cancer Investigation* 28: 4 (May 2010): 357-63.

33 Caffarel, Maria M, et al., "Cannabinoids reduce ErbB2-driven breast cancer progression through Akt inhibition," *Molecular Cancer* 9 (July 22, 2010): 196.

34 Whyte, DA, et al., "Cannabinoids inhibit cellular respiration of human oral cancer cells," *Pharmacology* 85: 6 (2010): 328-335.

35 Ibid.

36 Ibid.

37 Liang, C., et al., "A Population-Based Case-Control Study of Marijuana Use and Head and Neck Squamous Cell Carcinoma," *Cancer Prevention Research* 2 (August 2009): 759-68.

Chapter 4

38 Eubanks, Lisa M., et al., "A Molecular Link Between the Active Component of Marijuana and Alzheimer's Disease Pathology," *Molecular Pharmacy* 3: 6 (2006): 773-777.

39 "Marijuana's Active Ingredient Shown to Inhibit Primary Marker of Alzheimer's Disease" Press Release, The Scripps Research Institute, (August 9, 2006).

40 Jeffrey, Susan, "Dimebon Disappoints: Is There Hope for a Novel Alzheimer's Agent?," *Medscape Medical News*, (March 12, 2010) www.medscape.com/viewarticle/718401 (accessed February, 2011)

41 "Latest Buzz: Marijuana May Slow Progression of Alzheimer's disease" Ohio State University Research News, October 18, 2006 researchnews.osu.edu/archive/maricaff.htm (accessed February, 2011)

42 "Can Marijuana help treat Alzheimer's disease?" ProCon.org, medicalmarijuana.procon.org/viewanswers.asp?questionID=000130 (accessed February, 2011)

43 Ibid.

44 Ibid.

45 Wenk, Gary, Ph.D "Maintaining Memories with Marijuana," *Psychology Today*, (July 14, 2010) www.psychologytoday.com/blog/your-brain-food/201007/maintaining-memories-marijuana (accessed February, 2011)

46 Ramirez, Belen G., et al., "Prevention of Alzheimer's Disease Pathology by Cannabinoids: Neuroprotection Mediated by blockade of Microglial Activation," *Neurobiology of Disease* 25 (February 23, 2005): 1904-1913.

47 Campbel, V.A., Gowran, A., "Alzheimer's disease; taking the edge off with cannabinoids?" *British Journal of Pharmacology* 152, (November, 2007): 655-662.

48 Walton, Dawn, "Marijuana megadose may build better brains, curb depression and anxiety, study suggests," *The Globe and Mail*, Toronto, (October 14, 2005).

49 Jiang, W., et al., "Cannabinoids promote embryonic and adult hippocampus neurogenesis and produce anxiolytic- and antidepressant-like effects," *Journal of Clinical Investigation* 115 (November 2005): 3104-3116.

50 Shermer, Michael, "When Scientists Sin," *Scientific American* (July, 2010): 34.

51 Chen, b. et al., "Effect of Synthetic Cannabinoid HU210 on Memory Deficits and Neuropathology in Alzheimer's Disease Mouse Model," *Current Alzheimer Research* 7 (May 2010): 255-261.

52 "Marijuana doesn't help Alzheimer's disease," UPI.com (February 10, 2010). www.upi.com/Health_News/2010/02/10/Marijuana-doesnt-help-Alzheimers-disease/UPI-80781265844282/ (accessed February, 2011)

53 Croxford, J.L., "Therapeutic potential of cannabinoids in CNS disease," *CNS Drugs* 17 (2003): 179-202.

54 Hampson, A.J., et al., "Cannabidiol and delta-9-THC are neuroprotective antioxidants," *Medical Sciences* 95 (April 27, 1998): 8268-8273.

55 van der Stelt, M., et al., "Neuroprotection by delta-9-tetrahydrocannabinol, the Main Active Ingredient in Marijuana, against Ouabain-Induced in Vivo Excitotoxicity," *Journal of Neuroscience* (September 1, 2001): 6475-6479.

56 Ibid.

57 Mechoulam, Raphael, et al., "Endocannabinoids and Neuroprotection," *Science* 2002 (April 23, 2002): p.re5.

58 Mechoulam, Raphael, et al., "Cannabinoids and brain injury: therapeutic implications," *Trends in Molecular Medicine* 8: 2 (February, 2002): 58-61.

59 Gladwell, Malcolm "Offensive Play" *The New Yorker* (October 19, 2009).

60 Ibid.

61 Cabral, G.A., et al., "Cannabinoids as therapeutic agents for ablating neuroinflammatory disease," *Endocrin Metabolism Immune Disorder Drug Targets* 8 (September, 2008): 159-172.

62 Baker, David, Pryce, Gareth, "The therapeutic potential of cannabis in multiple sclerosis," *Expert Opinion on Investigational Drugs* 12 (April, 2003): 561-567.

63 Pate, David W. "Alternative Delivery Systems: Anandamides and Glaucoma" *National Conference on Cannabis Therapeutics*, (May 3-4, 2002, Portland, Oregon).

64 Shoemaker, Jenifer L., et al., "The CB2 cannabinoid agonist AM-1241 prolongs survival in a transgenic mouse model of amyotrophic lateral sclerosis," *Journal of Neurochemistry* 101(April, 2007): 87-98.

65 Carter, GT, et al., "Cannabis and Amyotrophic Lateral Sclerosis: Hypothetical and Practical Applications, and a Call for Clinical Trials." *American Journal of Hospital Palliative Care* (May 3, 2010).

66 Jacobus, J., et al., "White matter integrity in adolescents with histories of marijuana use and binge drinking," *Neurotoxicology and Teratology* 31 (November-December, 2009): 349-55.

67 Ellison, Katherine, "Medical Marijuana: No Longer Just for Adults," The *New York Times* (November 22, 2009).

68   Bergreen, Laurence, *Louis Armstrong: an Extravagant Life* (New York, Broadway Books, 1997): 284.

69   Ibid.

70   Ganon-Elazar, Eti, et al., "Cannabinoid Receptor Activation in the Basolateral Amygdala Blocks the Effects of Stress on the Conditioning and Extinction of Inhibitory Avoidance," *Journal of Neuroscience* 29 (Sept. 9, 2009): 11078-11088.

71   Tasker, Jeffrey, "Endogenous Cannabinoids Take the Edge off Neuroendocrine Responses to Stress", *Endocrinology* 145: 12 (2004): 5429-5430.

72   Massa, F., et al., "Endocannabinoids and the gastrointestinal tract," *Journal of Endocrinological Investigation* 29: 3supplement (2006): 47-57.

Chapter 5

73   Russo, Ethan and Guy, Geoffrey, "A Tale of Two Cannabinoids," *Medical Hypotheses* 66 (2006): 234-246.

74   Weiss, L. et al., "Cannabidiol arrests onset of autoimmune diabetes in NOD mice," *Neuropharmacology* 54: 1 (January 2008): 244-9.

75   Ibid.

76   Rajesh, Mohanraj, et al., "Cannabidiol Attenuates Cardiac Dysfunction, Oxidative Stress, Fibrosis and Inflammatory and Cell Death Signaling Pathways in Diabetic Cardiomyopathy," *Journal of the American College of Cardiology*, 56 (2010): 2115-2125.

77   Izzo, Angelo A., et al., "Non-psychotropic plant cannabinoids: new therapeutic opportunities from an ancient herb," *Trends in Pharmacological Sciences*, vol. 30 no. 10 (September, 2009): 515-527.

78   Mechoulam, R., et al., "Cannabidiol—Recent Advances," *Chemistry and Biodiversity* 4: 8 (August, 2007): 1678-1692.

79   Baker, Toni, "Compound found in marijuana may defend against diabetic retinopathy," *Medical College of Georgia—Science/Medical News* (February 27, 2006).

80   Gardner, Fred, "Mechoulam on Cannabidiol," *O'Shaughnessy's* (Winter/Spring 2008): 31.

81   McAllister, Sean, et al., "Cannabidiol as a novel inhibitor of Id-1 gene expression in aggressive breast cancer cells," *Molecular Cancer Therapeutics* 6 (November, 2007): 2121.

82   Gardner, Fred, "Studies Confirm Beneficial Effects of CBD, Terpenes," *O'Shaughnessy's* (Winter/Spring, 2008): 29.

83   www.projectcbd.com (accessed February, 2011)

84   Gardener, Fred. "Doctors to Study Effectiveness of CBD," *O'Shaughnessy's: The Journal of Cannabis in Clinical Practice*, Summer 2010: 41.

85 Gould, MN, "Cancer chemoprevention and therapy by monoterpenes," *Environmental Health Perspectives* 105: Suppl 4 (June, 1997): 977-979.

86 Crowell, PL, "Prevention and therapy of cancer by dietary monoterpenes," *Journal of Nutrition* 129(3) (March, 1999): 775S-778S.

87 Hazekamp, Arno, et al., "Biological activities of terpenoids," in Comprehensive Natural Products II Chemistry and Biology, vol.3, edited by Lew Mander and H. W. Lui (Oxford: Elsevier): 1061.

88 Ibid.

89 Stauth, David, "Studies force new view on biology of flavonoids," Press release, Oregon State University (March 5, 2007).

90 Ibid.

91 McPartland, John M. and Mediavilla, Vitto, "Noncannabinoid Components" in *Cannabis and Cannabinoids*, Grotenhemen MD, Franjo and Russo MD, Ethan, editors (The Haworth Integrative Healing Press, New York, 2002): 405.

Chapter 6

92 "Diet Drug Acomplia/Zimulti Dealt Blow as FDA Panel Says Keep It Off U.S. Market," *Zimulti Acomplia News*, (June, 2007). www.acompliareport.com/News/news-061807.htm (accessed February, 2011)

93 Ibid.

94 "Turned-off cannabinoid receptor turns on colorectal tumor growth," University of Texas M.D. Anderson Cancer Center, Press Release (August 1, 2008).

95 www.interpol.int/Public/Drugs/cannabis/default.asp (accessed February, 2011)

96 Roser, Patrick, "Antidepressant Effects of Cannabinoids," presentation at the 5th International Association for Cannabis as Medicine Conference, (October, 2009, Cologne , Germany).

97 Zimmer, A., et al., "Increased mortality, hypoactivity, and hypoalegesia in cannabinoids CB1 receptor knockout mice," *Proceedings of the National Academy of Sciences* 96, (May 11, 1999): 5780-5785.

98 Ibid.

99 Russo, Ethan B., "Clinical Endocannabinoid Deficiency (CECD): Can this Concept Explain Therapeutic Benefits of Cannabis in Migraine, Fibromyalgia, Irritable Bowel Syndrome and other Treatment-Resistant Conditions?," *Neuroendocrinology* Letters 25 (February-April, 2004): 31-39.

100 Ibid.

Chapter7

101   Russo, Ethan et al., "Phytochemical and Genetic Analyses of Ancient Cannabis from Central Asia," *Journal of Experimental Botany* 59: 15 (2008): 4171-4182.

102   Phalen, J.M., "The Marihuana Bugaboo," *Military Surgeon* 93 (1943): 94-95.

103   Gardner, Fred, "Notes for a Biography," *O'Shaughnessy's* (Winter/Spring, 2008): 16.

Chapter 8

104   Mechoulam, Raphael, "Journal Interview 85," *Addiction* 102: 6 (2007): 887-893.

105   Grinspoon, Lester, *Marihuana Reconsidered*, (Oakland, CA: Quick American Archives, 1994): vii.

106   Ibid.

107   Weil, Andrew, "What No One Wants to Know", *The Natural Mind*, (New York: Houghton Mifflin, 1986): 74.

108   Ibid., 81.

109   "Studying the Effects of Marijuana," youtube video, www.youtube.com/watch?v=uw85USZt6Dg (accessed February, 2011).

110   Statement of Leo E. Hollister, M.D., Medical Investigator, Veterans Administration Hospital, before Congress (1970): 1.

111   Baum, Dan, "Pee House of the August Moon," *Smoke and Mirrors*, (Boston, Little, Brown and Company, 1996): 63.

112   National Commission on Marihuana and Drug Abuse, *Marihuana: A Signal of Misunderstanding*, U.S. Government Printing Office (1972, Washington, D.C.): 23.

113   Ibid., 140.

114   Ibid., 152.

115   "President Richard M. Nixon's 23rd News Conference" (March 24, 1972, Washington, D.C).

116   *Marihuana: A Signal of Misunderstanding.* p. 176.

Chapter 9

117   Munson, A.E., et al., "Anticancer Activity of Cannabinoids," *Journal of the National Cancer Institute* 55, (September 1975): 597.

118   Randall, Robert, O'Leary, Alice, *Marijuana Rx: The Patients' fight for Medicinal Pot*, (New York: Thunder's Mouth Press, 1998): 108.

119   Ibid., 278.

Chapter 11

120 Gottlieb, M.S., et al., "Pneumocystis Pneumonia—Los Angeles," *Morbidity and Mortality Weekly Report* (June 5, 1981): 11.

121 New Mexico State Department of Health, "Oral Vs. Inhaled cannabinoids for Nausea/ Vomiting from Cancer Chemotherapy" (November, 1986).

122 Joy, Janet, et al., editors, *Marijuana and Medicine: Assessing the Science Base* (Washington, D.C., National Academy Press, 1999): 203.

123 Kevin Zeese, personal communication, John Morgan, personal communication.

124 Mack, Alison and Joy, Janet, *Marijuana As Medicine?* (Washington, D.C.: National Academy Press, 2001): 144.

125 Kevin Zeese, personal communication (1997).

126 *In the Matter of Marijuana Rescheduling, Docket 86-22, Opinion, Recommended Ruling, Findings of Fact, Conclusions of Law, and Decision of Administrative Law Judge,* (Washington, D.C,: Drug Enforcement Administration, September 6, 1988) and personal communication with Kevin Zeese.

127 *In the Matter of Marijuana Rescheduling.*

128 Ibid.

129 Randall, Robert, and O'Leary: 295.

130 Randall, R.C., *Marijuana and AIDS: Pot, Politics and PWAs in America* (Washington, DC: Galen Press, 1991): 66.

Chapter 12

131 Randall, Robert, and O'Leary: 327.

132 Ibid., 359-360.

133 Doblin, RE and Kleiman, Mark, "Medical Use of Marijuana," *Annals of Internal Medicine* 114 (May, 1991): 809-810.

134 Isikoff, Michael, "HHS to phase out marijuana program," *Washington Post* (June 22, 1991): A14.

135 Randall, Robert and O'Leary: 25.

136 TODAY Show transcript, NBC (May 6, 1991): 25.

137 Ostrow, R., "Delay in lifting pot ban to seriously ill is assailed," *Los Angeles Times* (January 31, 1992): A13.

Chapter 13

138 Peron, Dennis, personal communication (1996).

139 Plasse, Terry et al., "Dronabinol Stimulates Appetite and Weight Gain in HIV Patients," 8: 122, (PuB 7442), *VII International Conference on AIDS* (July, 1992).

140   Leshner, A., Letter to Donald Abrams (1995).

141   Abrams, D.I., Letter to Alan Leshner, NIDA (1995).

Chapter 14

142   Public Law 92-255, *National Institute on Drug Abuse: National Council on Drug Abuse* (1972): 55.

143   Abrams, D.I., "Medical marijuana: Tribulations and trials," *Journal of Psychoactive Drugs* 30: 2 (1998): 166.

144   Russell, S., "U.S. Drug Czar Visits Haight, denounces medical use of pot," *San Francisco Chronicle* (Aug. 16, 1996): A8.

145   Kanigal, R., "Medical marijuana heads for the Nov. 5 battlefield," *Oakland Tribune* (October 20, 1996): C1.

146   Barry McCaffrey, et al., press conference, *CNN* (December 30, 1996).

147   Doblin, R. fax to Donald Abrams (1997).

148   Abrams, D.I., personal communication (1997).

Chapter 15

149   Joy, Janet E.: 177.

150   Ibid., 179.

Chapter 16

151   Abrams, Donald I., et al., "Short-term effects of cannabinoids in patients with HIV-1 infection: a randomized, placebo-controlled clinical trial," *Annals of Internal Medicine*, 139: 4 (August 19, 2003): 258-265.

152   "Marijuana does not appear to alter viral loads of HIV patients taking protease inhibitors," UCSF News Office (July 13, 2000). news.ucsf. edu/releases/marijuana-does-not-appear-to-alter-viral-loads-of-hiv-patients-taking-prote/ (accessed February, 2011).

153   "UCSF Study Finds No Harm to HIV Positive Patients With Short-Term Medical Cannabis," UCSF Press Release (Aug. 18, 2003). www. maps.org/mmj/ucsfpr8.18.03.html (accessed February, 2011).

154   Nahas, G. and Pace N. "Marijuana Smoking As Medicine: a Cruel Hoax," New York University Medical Center (2000). www.druglibrary. org/Schaffer/hemp/medical/mjhoax.htm (accessed February, 2011).

155   "Despite Marijuana Furor, 8 Users Get Drug From Government," *New York Times,* (December 1, 1996).

156   Russo, E. et al., "Chronic Cannabis Use in the Compassionate Investigational New Drug Program: an Examination of Benefits and Adverse Effects of Legal Cannabis," *Journal of Cannabis Therapeutics* 2: 1 (2002): 3-55.

Chapter 17

157   Abrams, D. et al., "Vaporization as a Smokeless Cannabis Delivery System: a Pilot Study," *Clinical Pharmacology and Therapeutics* 82 (November, 2007): 572-578.

158   Aggarwal, Sunil K. et al., "Medicinal use of cannabis in the United States: Historical perspectives, current trends, and future directions," *Journal of Opiod Management* 5 (May/June, 2009): 153-167.

159   Grinspoon, Lester and Bakalar, James B., *Marihuana: The Forbidden Medicine* (New Haven, Connecticut, Yale University Press: 1993): 12-13.

160   American Medical Association Board of Trustee and Council Reports-Recommendations (2009): 14.

161   Hoeffel, John, "Medical Marijuana Gets Boost from Major Doctors' Group," *Los Angeles Times* (November 11, 2009).

162   "American College of Physicians. Supporting Research into the Therapeutic Role of Marijuana," American College of Physicians, Position Paper," Philadelphia (2008).

Chapter 18

163   NIDA Research Report Series-Marijuana Abuse, www.virginia.edu/case/ATOD/RRMarijuana.pdf (accessed February, 2011).

164   Ibid.

165   Swerdlow, Lanny, "Dr. Donald Tashkin Marijuana Lung Cancer Study Pt. 1 of 2," youtube interview with Donald Tashkin. www.youtube.com/watch?v=GJmQ16cGBHU (accessed February 2011)

166   NIDA.

167   Vinson, D., "Marijuana and other illicit drug use and the risk of injury: a case-controlled study," *Missouri Medicine* 103: 2 (2006).

168   Gmel, Gerhard, et al., "Alcohol and cannabis use as risk factors for injury—a case-crossover analysis in a Swiss hospital emergency department," *BMC Public Health* 9, (2009)

169   FDA Briefing Document, "NDA 21-888, Zimulti (rimonabant) Tablets 20 mg. Sanofi Aventis Advisory Committee," (June 13, 2007): 35.

170   Ibid.

171   NIDA.

172   Mechoulam, Raphael, "The Cannabinoid System in Neuroprotection," lecture at Third National Clinical Conference Cannabis Therapeutics, Charlottesville,VA (May, 2004). www.youtube.com/watch?v=Wmqh1Q2cnD0 (accessed February, 2011)

173   Setoodeh, Ramin, "Smith's Newest Jones" *Newsweek* (June 11, 2009). www.newsweek.com/2009/06/10/smith-s-newest-jones.html# (accessed February, 2011)

174   Lyketsos, Constantine G.., "Cannabis Use and Cognitive Decline in Persons under 65 Years of Age," *American Journal of Epidemiology* 149: 9 (May 1, 1999): 794-800.

175   Haney, Margaret, et al., "Dronabinol and Marijuana in HIV-Positive Marijuana Sokers: Caloric Intake, Mood and Sleep," *JAIDS: Journal of Acquired Immune Deficiency Syndromes* 45 (August, 2007): 545-554.

176   Time.com "Top 10 Non-Emergency 911 Calls." www.time.com/time/specials/packages/article/0,28804,1903486_1903487_1903417,00.html (accessed February 2011)

177   "Marijuana's Potency Has Increased Over Time," U.S. Department of Health and Human Services, Substance Abuse and Mental Health Services Administration, Family Guide (2004).

178   Andreasson, S., et al., "Cannabis and schizophrenia. A longitudinal study of Swedish conscripts," *Lancet* 2 (December, 1987): 1483-6.

179   Zimmer, Lynn, Ph.D., Morgan, John P., *Marijuana Myths/Marijuana Facts*, (New York: Lindesmith Center, 1997): 82.

180   "Brown Says Message Must Be Sent on Cannabis," *Reuters UK* (April 30, 2008).

181   David Nutt, interview, Skynews, November 2, 2009, www.youtube.com/watch?v=bCChf2WHNE4&feature=PlayList&p=2AD9B115E7FAB525&playnext=1&playnext_from=PL&index=1 (accessed February, 2011)

182   Gardner, Fred, "Cannabis and Schizophrenia," *O'Shaughnessy's* (Winter/Spring, 2008): 34.

183   Ibid.

184   Macleod, John, "Psychological and social sequelae of cannabis and other illicit drug use by young people: a systematic review of longitudinal, general population studies," *The Lancet* 363: 9421 (May 15, 2004): 1578-1588.

185   Colin Blakemore, Ph.D., e-mail to ProCon.org, (December 27, 2002). medicalmarijuana.procon.org/view.answers.php?questionID=000220 (accessed February, 2011).

186   Frisher, Martin, et al., "Assessing the impact of cannabis use on trends in diagnosed schizophrenia in the United Kingdom from 1996 to 2005," *Schizophrenia Research* 113 (September, 2009): 123-128.

187   Schwarcz, G., Karajgi B., et al., "Synthetic delta-9-tetrahydrocannabinol (dronabinol) can improve the symptoms of schizophrenia," *Journal of Clinical Psychopharmacology* 29 (June, 2009): 255-8.

188   Leweke, F.M., et al., "S30-02 Antipsychotic effects of cannabidiol," *Psychopharmacology* 142 (March 1999): 230-235.

189   "Growing Evidence of Marijuana Smoke's Potential Dangers," *Science Daily* (August 5, 2009) www.sciencedaily.com/releases/ 2009/08/090805110741.htm (accessed February, 2011)

190   Ibid.

191   Tashkin, Donald, "Does Regular Marijuana Smoking Lead to Pulmonary Disease (COPD, lung cancer, pneumonia)?," lecture, Fifth National Clinical Conference on Cannabis Therapeutics, Asilomar, California (April, 2008).

192   Bambico, Francis Rodriguez, et al., "Cannabis Damages Young Brains More than Originally Thought, Study Finds," *Science Daily* (December 20, 2009) www.sciencedaily.com/releases/2009/12/091217115834.htm (accessed February, 2011).

193   Barbeau, Bernard, "Cannabis brain damage worse in teens than thought," (December 18, 2009). www.healthzone.ca/health/article/740642 (accessed February, 2011).

194   Blanchard RN, Kathleen, "Cannabis is more damaging to adolescent brains than previously known," emaxhealth.com (December 18, 2009). www.emaxhealth.com/1020/22/34829/cannabis-more-damaging-adolescent-brains-previously-known.html (accessed February, 2011).

195   NIDA Research Report Series-Marijuana Abuse (2008). www.zgxl.net/ eng/health/addiction/marijuana.htm (accessed February, 2011)

196   Harris, Gardiner, "Researchers find study of medical marijuana discouraged," *New York Times* (January 19, 2010): A14.

197   Haney, Margret, et al., "Dronabinol and Marijuana in HIV-Positive Marijuana Smokers: Caloric Intake, Mood, and Sleep," *JAIDS: Journal of Acquired Immune Deficiency Syndromes* 45 (August, 2007): 545-554.

198   Marcu, Jahan P. et al., "Cannabidiol Enhances the Inhibitory Effects of delta-9-Tetrahydrocannabinol on Human Glioblastoma Cell Proliferation and Survival," *Molecular Cancer Therapeutics* 9 (January, 2010): 180-189.

199   Joy, Janet, *Marijuana and Medicine*, 100-101.

200   Zimmer, Lynn, Morgan, John, 37.

201   Menetrey, A., et al., "Assessment of driving capability through the use of clinical and psychomotor tests in relation to blood cannabinoid levels following oral administration of 20 mg dronabinol or of a cannabis decoction made with 20 and 60mg delta-9-THC," *Journal of Analytical Toxicology* 29(2005): 327-338.

202   U.S. Department of Transportation, National Highway Traffic Safety
      Administration. *State of Knowledge of Drugged Driving: FINAL RE-
      PORT* (September, 2003).

203   Marijuana Abuse, Research Report Series, 2005, NIDA web page.
      www.drugabuse.gov/ResearchReports/Marijuana/Marijuana5.
      html#treatments (accessed December, 2009).

204   Levine, Harry G. "New York's Marijuana Arrest Crusade—Con-
      tinues," (September 2009): 8. www.ssc.wisc.edu/~wright/125-2010/
      NYC-MARIJUANA-ARREST-CRUSADE-CONTINUES-FEB-2010.
      pdf (accessed February, 2011).

205   Ibid., 9.

Chapter 19

206   Block, RI, et al., "Effects of chronic marijuana use on testosterone,
      luteinizing hormone, follicle stimulating hormone, prolactin and cor-
      tisol in men and women," *Drug and Alcohol Dependence* 28 (August,
      1991): 121-8.

207   Hembree, W.C. et al., "Changes in Human Spermatozoa Associated
      with High Dose Marihuana Smoking," in *Marihuana: Biological Ef-
      fects*, Nahas, G.G. and Paton, W.D.M., editors (Oxford: Pergamon Press,
      1979): 429-439.

208   Zygmunt, M., et al., "Angiogenesis and vasculogenesis in pregnancy,"
      European Journal of Obstetrics, Gynecology and Reproductive Biology
      110 (September, 2003): S10-8.

209   Ness, Roberta B., et al., "Cocaine and Tobacco Use and the Risk of
      Spontaneous Abortion," *The New England Journal of Medicine*, 340: 5
      (February 4, 1999): 333-339.

210   National Toxicology Project Report, THC p. 41.

211   Bambico, F.R. et al., "Chronic exposure to cannabinoids during adoles-
      cence but not during adulthood impairs emotional behavior and mono-
      aminergic neurotransmission," *Neurobiological Disease* 37 (March
      2010): 641-655.

212   Liang, C., et al.

Chapter 20

213   BJS, "Scientists find organic farms have higher quality fruit, better
      soil, lower environmental impact," Science Blog (September 2, 2010).
      scienceblog.com/38109/scientists-find-organic-farms-have-higher-
      quality-fruit-better-soil-lower-environmental-impact/ (accessed Feb-
      ruary, 2011).

214 "Stiletto Stoners," *TODAY Show* (October 1, 2009). www.youtube.com/watch?v=J3ODIhXC0IY (accessed February, 2011)

215 Wenk, *Maintaining Memories.*

216 Ibid.

217 Ibid.

218 "Increasing Substance Abuse Levels among Older Adults Likely to Create Sharp Rise in Need for Treatment Services in Next Decade," SAMHSA News Release (January 8, 2010).

219 SAMHSA News Release, Increasing Substance Abuse Levels.

220 NIDA Research Report Series-Marijuana Abuse.

221 NIDA Info Facts, National Institute on Drug Abuse, drugabuse.gov/infofacts/marijuana.html (accessed February, 2011)

222 Wenk, *Maintaining Memories.*

ACKNOWLEDGMENTS

M Y THANKS AND DEEPEST APPRECIATION to: Donald—because I could not have done this, or so many other things, without you. Pete Masterson—author of *Book Design and Production,* my designer and primary guide in this self-publishing effort, it's great working with the best! Brad Burge—for doing such a beautiful job of editing my work. Lin Lacombe of Communications Consultants—for helping me to get the word out about my book. Chris Merritt—for designing my web site and easing me into the 21st Century. J. Naomi Linzer—for indexing my book thoroughly. Shelley Lazar—because you're the Queen of Joy. Marsha Rosenbaum, Ph.D.—for proofreading, input and cheerleading. Rick Doblin, Ph.D.—for founding MAPS and pointing me to Brad Burge. Ethan Russo, M.D. —for answering my questions immediately. Manuel Guzman, Ph.D.—for answering my questions so well. Valerie Corral—for being you. Dennis Peron—for giving me complete access to the Cannabis Buyers' Club to interview employees and patients. Fred Gardner—for your scholarship and advice. Al Byrne and Mary Lynn Mathre—for founding Patients Out of Time and putting on the conferences where I learned so much. Keith Stroup—for founding the National Organization for the Reform of Marijuana Laws (NORML) and taking time to encourage me. Alan St. Pierre—for working so hard with NORML and giving me my first public speaking opportunity. David Bienenstock—for asking me to speak at the High Times Medical Cannabis Cup. Paul Armentano—a fellow science scribe, friend and sounding board. Dale Gieringer, Ph.D.—for running California NORML and doing exceptional research. Michelle and Michael Aldrich—for so many things, but specifically, for eagle-eye proofreading.

I also want to thank the following people for encouraging me, assisting me and/or informing me: Debby Goldsberry, Angel Raiche, Angela Fairless, The research librarians at the San Francisco Public Library, Jeff Jones, Steve Ellis, M.D., Jorge Cervantes, Marcia Degelman, Joan Kirsch, the members of the Bay Area Independent Publishers Association, David Nick, Tony Serra, Marcus Conant, M.D., the team at Steep Hill Laboratories, Kara Brown, Uncle George and Aunt Winnie, Ellen Kaufman, Lenore Leach, Connie and Gary, Wendy and Maggie Serenity, Storm I.B., Linda O', Charlotte, Taffe and Bill, Tomoko, Luke, Danni, Connor, Zoe, and Lanny, Josh at Drewe's Brothers' Meats in San Francisco, Paul and Barbara, Irv Rosenfeld, author of My Medicine, Alice O'Leary, Anna Boyce, Reverend Joey, Jerry and Diane, Betty Lamb, Sidney Stafford, and thank you to the Hemperor Jack Herer, for writing *The Emperor Wears No Clothes* a book that changed the world.

ABOUT THE AUTHOR

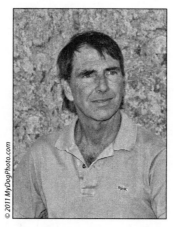

CLINT WERNER HAS DEGREES IN journalism and library science and has worked in the field of preventive health for over 25 years. His writing has appeared in *Cannabis Therapeutics in HIV/AIDS*, the *Journal of Cannabis Therapeutics*, *Macrobiotics Today*, *Canine Chronicle*, and other publications.

INDEX

CPSIA information can be obtained at www.ICGtesting.com
Printed in the USA
LVOW092029120212

268299LV00003B/1/P